Case Presentations in Urology

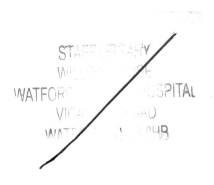

Presented with the co.

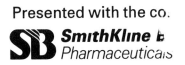

SmithKline b
Pharmaceuticals

Titles in the series

Case Presentations in Urology

P. Abrams MD FRCS
Consultant Urologist, Bristol Urological Institute
Southmead Hospital, Westbury-on-Trym, Bristol

R. C. L. Feneley MChir FRCS
Consultant Urologist, Bristol Urological Institute
Southmead Hospital, Westbury-on-Trym, Bristol

D. A. Gillatt ChM FRCS
Consultant Urologist, Bristol Urological Institute
Southmead Hospital, Westbury-on-Trym, Bristol

J. C. Gingell FRCS
Consultant Urologist, Bristol Urological Institute
Southmead Hospital, Westbury-on-Trym, Bristol

J. D. Frank FRCS
Consultant Paediatric Urologist, Bristol Urological Institute
Southmead Hospital, Westbury-on-Trym, Bristol
and Bristol Royal Hospital for Sick Children

A. Hinchliffe ChM FRCS
Consultant Urologist, Bristol Urological Institute
Southmead Hospital, Westbury-on-Trym, Bristol
and Weston General Hospital, Weston-super-Mare

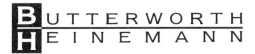

Butterworth-Heinemann Ltd
Linacre House, Jordan Hill, Oxford OX2 8DP

ℛ A member of the Reed Elsevier group

OXFORD   LONDON   BOSTON
MUNICH   NEW DELHI   SINGAPORE   SYDNEY
TOKYO   TORONTO   WELLINGTON

First published 1993
Reprinted 1994

British Library Cataloguing in Publication Data
Abrams, Paul
    Case Presentations in Urology. – (Case
    Presentation Series)
    I. Title II. Series
    616.6

ISBN 0 7506 0527 8

Library of Congress Cataloguing in Publication Data
Case presentations in urology/Paul Abrams . . . [et al.].
    p. cm. – (Case presentations series)
    Includes bibliographical references and index.
    ISBN 0 7506 0527 8
    1. Genitourinary organs – Diseases – Case studies. 2. Urology –
    Case studies. I. Abrams, Paul, 1947–. II. Series.
    [DNLM: 1. Urologic Diseases – case studies. WJ 100 C3365 1993]
    RC877.C37   1993
    616.6'09–dc20   93–30540
                                                                CIP

Typeset by BC Typesetting, Warmley, Bristol BS15 5YD
Printed in Great Britain at the University Press, Cambridge

Paediatric urology

Case 1

A 24-year-old primgravida had a routine prenatal ultrasound scan performed at 30 weeks of gestation. An incidental finding was moderate dilatation of the kidneys bilaterally and a thick walled full bladder that failed to empty on subsequent examinations. The fetus was a male infant confirmed by visualization of the genitalia.

Questions

1 What is the most likely diagnosis?
2 How should the situation be managed?

Answers

1 The likely cause of this abnormality in a male fetus is bladder outlet obstruction due to a posterior urethral valve. The differential diagnosis includes bilateral pelvi-ureteric junction obstruction or bilateral obstructive mega-ureters, but the bladder in these patients is normal and is seen on ultrasound to empty normally. Prune belly syndrome is associated with gross bilateral hydro-nephrosis and a megacystis in which the bladder is not thick walled. If the prune belly syndrome is severe, oligo-hydramnios may be noted and the degree of hydro-nephrosis is normally much greater than in a patient with valves.
2 The rest of the pregnancy will have to be followed closely by serial ultrasounds. These are to monitor the degree of upper tract dilatation and whether or not any oligo-hydramnios develops. Progressive oligohydramnios with

an apparently obstructed bladder associated with kidneys with reasonable renal tissue picked up after 20 weeks' gestation is probably one of the few indications for a percutaneous prenatal vesico-amniotic shunt. This particular child did not develop oligohydramnios and was born spontaneously at 39 weeks' gestation.

Routine postnatal examination was unremarkable. The bladder was noted to be palpable and the infant was seen to have a poor stream. Antibiotics were started. Postnatal ultrasound confirmed bilateral hydronephrosis, worse on the left side than the right, together with a distended thick walled bladder and dilated posterior urethra. There was good preservation of renal cortex on the right side but thin cortex on the left. Renal function was normal. A cystogram was performed which showed a classic urethral valve with gross reflux up the left ureter. The child was left catheterized. The following day he was taken to theatre and a Type I urethral valve was resected using an infant 10F resectoscope. Postoperatively the child was catheterized for 24 hours. The catheter was removed and the child was discharged home well with normal renal function 3 days after surgery. Two months after surgery a DMSA scan showed no function of the left kidney but a normal right kidney. Cystogram confirmed gross reflux up the left ureter and with good evidence of fulgaration of the valve on the voiding views of the urethra. Because of the non-functioning grossly refluxing left system, a left nephro-ureterectomy was performed at 6 months of age. The child has remained well and normal since then.

A posterior urethral valve (Figure 1) is an uncommon congenital abnormality seen in between 1:5000–6000 live male births. More of these patients are now being diagnosed antenatally because of routine antenatal ultrasound screening. Those fetuses who are found to have gross bilateral hydronephrosis and oligohydramnios before 20 weeks' gestation normally have such severe renal damage that a termination of pregnancy is probably indicated. Those patients who have less severe oligohydramnios diagnosed after 20 weeks' gestation may occasionally benefit from a vesicoamniotic shunt, but the initial enthusiasm for this procedure has now calmed down. Only occasionally is a patient suitable for this type of treatment. After delivery if a baby is preterm or small a temporary vesi-

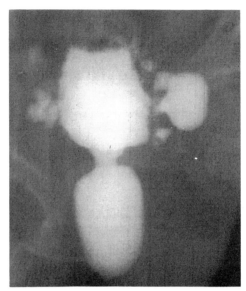

Figure 1 X-ray showing posterior urethral valve

costomy should be performed as attempts at instrumentation of a neonatal urethra may lead to long-term damage and stricture formation. Providing the infant is of normal gestation and of a good size a 10 French resectoscope can be safely used. Fifty per cent of patients with valves reflux and 50% of these will eventually ceased spontaneously. Nephroureterectomy is indicated for non-function and reflux, but there is little indication for other major surgery. In those patients with compromised renal function and a significantly hypocompliant bladder, augmentation may be required. Improvement in early mortality, which has occurred in recent years, has been offset by the increase in long-term morbidity with more patients going into renal failure and requiring transplantation.

Case 2

A routine maternal ultrasound scan at 20 weeks' gestation showed that an apparently normal fetus had a dilated left renal pelvis.

4

Questions

1   What is the antenatal management of this patient?
2   How should the infant be managed after birth?

Answers

1   During the initial assessment of this fetus by ultrasound a number of questions need to be answered.

    a   Is the fetus male or female?
    b   Is the bladder normal?
    c   Are the ureters normal?
    d   Is the hydronephrosis unilateral or bilateral?

This child was male because of identification of a normal penis and therefore it is important that a diagnosis of urethral valves is excluded. There was no oligohydramnios and the bladder was seen to fill and empty normally. The bladder was not thick walled and therefore a diagnosis of valves can almost certainly be excluded. The hydro-nephrosis was noted to be unilateral and the ureters were not visualized. A presumptive diagnosis therefore of a left pelviureteric junction obstruction was made. The abnormality was discussed with the parents. It was explained that it was unilateral and that it was impossible to say whether or not the baby would require postnatal surgery. Whether surgery was required or not the prognosis was excellent. The parents therefore agreed to continue with the pregnancy.

The fetus was monitored with regular ultrasound estimations every 4 weeks. These confirmed a persisting hydronephrosis, but the other kidney remained normal. The baby was born normally at 39 weeks' gestation by vaginal delivery. Postnatal examination revealed a healthy 3 kg infant with no obvious abnormalities.

2   A postnatal ultrasound was performed on day 2 which confirmed a normal right kidney and a hydronephrotic left kidney with a large renal pelvis. Not infrequently when babies are born who have had a minor degree of hydro-nephrosis prenatally, postnatal examination reveals apparently normal kidneys. This is probably due to the fact that urine flow rates are highest during the last trimester of

pregnancy. In this baby the hydronephrosis persisted. Further investigations are therefore required to determine whether the kidney is significantly obstructed and whether surgery is required. Prior to discharge from hospital a micturating cystogram was performed which showed a normal male urethra with no reflux. The baby was therefore discharged with antibiotic prophylaxis for further investigations to be undertaken.

The investigation required is an isotope renogram. Because the neonatal kidney is immature and maturation of glomerular and tubular function has not occurred it is best to wait until after the transitional phase of nephrology is finished before undertaking the investigations. We would therefore normally investigate the child at approximately 4 weeks of age.

A renogram is best undertaken using Mag 3. Considerable controversy exists as to what constitutes an obstructed kidney and even more so when one is talking about an obstructed neonatal kidney. Some authors consider the percentage of overall renal function to be important, others consider the uptake curve, while others consider the excretion curves to be the most important. Occasionally, as in this child, one will get a suggestion from all three criteria that the kidney is obstructed, i.e. the left kidney contributed only 30% of overall renal function, the uptake and excretion curves were slow and there was no drainage after the administration of Lasix. Because of this the infant underwent a pyeloplasty at the age of 2 months when a routine Anderson-Hynes pyeloplasty was undertaken using loop magnification. Neither a nephrostomy nor ureteric stent were placed in situ and the baby made an uneventful postoperative recovery being discharged from hospital 3 days after the surgery. A follow-up renogram at 3 months showed improved drainage with a differential function of 40%. Prophylactic antibiotics have been discontinued.

If one is in doubt as to whether a kidney is obstructed in the neonatal period, i.e. it is functioning well with 50% of overall renal function, and the drainage slow after Lasix, we would not subject the baby to surgery but would re-investigate at 6 months of age with a further Mag 3 scan. If differential function is well maintained on the Mag 3 scan we would continue to follow the child conservatively. If function appeared to show deterioration or the child developed a urinary tract infection we would proceed to a pyeloplasty. It is more difficult to assess children who have a bilateral pelviureteric junction obstruction in this age group because one does not have a normal contralateral kidney with which to compare the drainage or the function. On the whole the key to management of these patients should be conservative unless there are major indications to intervene surgically.

Case 3

On routine examination of a baby in the postnatal ward 24 hours after a breach delivery a swollen left testis was found.

Questions

1 What is the most likely cause of this abnormality?
2 How would you manage such a patient?

Answers

1 The most likely diagnosis of a scrotal mass in the neonatal period is a perinatal torsion of the testis. The differential diagnosis is a hernia, a testicular tumour, a hydrocele or trauma to the testis following a difficult breach delivery. A careful clinical examination will help to differentiate the diagnosis together with the ultrasound. A perinatal torsion of the testis is diagnosed by finding a firm hard testis which appears to be non-tender. There is no swelling in the groin and the testis does not transilluminate.
2 A perinatal testicular torsion may occur prenatally or at delivery and the findings on examination do depend on the time at which the torsion has occurred. If the torsion has occurred around about the time of delivery there may be some erythema associated with a small hydrocele. A peri-natal testicular torsion is normally extravaginal because the tunica vaginalis has a normal insertion and the attach-ments between the tunica and the scrotum are flimsy, thus

allowing the whole of the scrotal content to twist around the cord.

By the time of diagnosis the testis is infarcted and it is not usually possible to salvage it. We would normally explore such a testis within the next 24 hours but not as a desperate emergency. Confirmation of the diagnosis is made by finding a black testis which is removed. The contralateral testis is fixed by carrying out a Jaboulay procedure and fixing it in a Dartos pouch without suture fixation. We fix all solitary testes so as to avoid the rare but serious consequences of undergoing a torsion of the second testis.

Case 4

On routine postnatal examination an apparently healthy male infant was noted to have a phallus of moderate size with chordee, a penoscrotal hypospadias and bilaterally impalpable testes.

Questions

1 What investigations should be performed?
2 How should the child be managed?

Answers

1 The most important diagnosis to avoid missing is that of the adreno-genital syndrome (congenital adrenal hyperplasia (CAH)). Too often babies with this diagnosis are thought of as males with severe hypospadias and discharged from hospital with an incorrect diagnosis. They may then present in the first few weeks of life, acutely unwell, with a salt-losing crisis. This is a serious complication and may lead to the death of the child.

These babies should therefore have their chromosomes analysed which will show a normal female karyotype of 46XX. Sixty per cent of intersex patients have CAH. Ninety per cent have a block in 21 hydroxylation. The two other types are a block of 11 hydroxylase or 3 beta hydroxysteroid dehydrogenase. The commonest form of CAH has an excess production of 17-hydroxyprogesterone and therefore plasma should be sent for analysis of the 17-hydroxyprogesterone level. The differential diagnosis is that of a male with a severe perineal hypospadias and bilateral intra-abdominal testes. Virilization of a normal female fetus due to maternal ingestion of androgens during pregnancy, which was seen not infrequently during the 1960s, is now rarely seen.

2   In this patient investigations revealed an elevated plasma level of 17-hydroxyprogesterone, normal electrolytes and a normal female karotype. The diagnosis of CAH was therefore confirmed. Having established this diagnosis the child was initially referred to a paediatric endocrinologist for medical management. She was stabilized on hydrocortisone and fluorocortisone because she was a salt loser. A urethrogram was performed to determine the entry site of the vagina into the urogenital sinus. The complexity of the surgery will be determined by whether the vaginal opening is high or low. If the vagina is not visualized on the X-ray, a cystoscopy will be required with the introduction of a retrograde catheter into the vagina and a vaginogram taken using contrast medium. These patients with severe virilization will usually have a high vaginal insertion into the urogenital sinus.

Surgery is normally undertaken when the medical condition of the child is stable. In the recent past a cliteroplasty to reduce the size of the clitoris was undertaken in the neonatal period so that the child had normal appearing genitalia on discharge from hospital. At the same time if the vaginal opening was low, a flap vaginoplasty was performed. If it was high a complex pull through vaginoplasty would be required and this was normally carried out at the age of 3–4 years. More recently Passerini has described an operation requiring the cliteroplasty and vaginoplasty be performed at the same time in a severely virilized female with a high vaginal opening. Both of these operations are performed when the child is a few months of age as a single stage procedure. In the past some surgeons have insisted that routine vaginal dilatations be performed after surgery until the child is adolescent. We have always felt that this is an unnecessary intrusion on the child and the parents and would prefer to do nothing until the child is nearing puberty. At this age an examination under anaesthesia is performed to assess the size of the vaginal opening prior to the use of tampons and intercourse. If the vaginal opening has narrowed, further surgery is undertaken to enlarge this opening and the teenager then uses regular vaginal dilatations until starting sexual intercourse. The child will require maintenance on steroids for the rest of her life and will be followed regularly by the paediatric endocrinologist who will monitor her steroid replacement requirements.

Reference

GIACOMO, PASSERINI and GLAZEL, 1989, A new one-stage procedure for clitero-vaginoplasty in severely mascularized female pseudohermaphrodites. *Journal of Urology*, **142**, 565–567

Case 5

On a routine postnatal examination an otherwise healthy young male infant was found to have an impalpable right testis. The left testis was normally descended.

Question

How should this infant be managed?

Answer

A baby with an undescended testis should be referred to the paediatric urological outpatient clinic at the age of 6 weeks.

This allows examination of the undescended testis to be undertaken prior to the cremasteric reflex becoming active. The diagnosis of descent and undescent can then be made more easily. Examination of this patient failed to reveal any evidence of a right testis either in the scrotum, the groin or the perineum. The finding of an impalpable testis was discussed with the mother at this time. There are three possible diagnoses. The testis may be present but either intra-abdominal or high up within the inguinal canal or the testis may be absent. The commonest cause for monorchia is a prenatal torsion of an intra-abdominal testis. The baby should be re-examined at 6 months of age to confirm that the testis remains impalpable as occasionally a high testis may descend spontaneously in the first few weeks of life.

On examination at the age of 9 months the testis was still impalpable. The contralateral testis appeared to be of a normal size for the age of the child. Patients with monorchia tend to undergo compensatory hypertrophy of the remaining testis. It has been reported that a testis that has a diameter greater than two standard deviations above the norm for the age suggests the contralateral testis is absent. This hypothesis requires further clinical confirmation.

This patient should have a laparoscopy to exclude or confirm the presence of an intra-abdominal testis. Methods used for localizing the testis in an adult such as ultrasound examination or a CT scan are not suitable for children and babies as the testis is too small to be picked up. Laparoscopy enables an intra-abdominal testis to be diagnosed or confirmation of monorchia made by finding blind-ending testicular vessels and a blind-ending vas on the side of the impalpable testis. If monorchia is confirmed on laparoscopy no further surgical procedure is required apart from fixation of the contralateral testis within a Dartos pouch to avoid the small but disastrous risk of a contralateral torsion. If, when the child goes through puberty, he is concerned about having only one testis it is reasonable to put in a silastic prosthesis. If an intra-abdominal testis is found it may either be removed or an orchidopexy performed. Many surgeons feel that as these testes are highly abnormal and dysgeneic they are better removed. If an orchidopexy is undertaken it is normally necessary to carry out a Fowler-Stephens orchidopexy with division of the testicular artery and vein with the reliance for the blood supply upon the peritoneal vessels and the artery to the vas.

If a baby only had one testis which was intra-abdominal it is better brought down using a microvascular technique with anastomosis between the testicular vessels and the inferior epigastric artery and vein.

Case 6

An 18-month-old child presented with lethargy, failure to thrive and generally unwell. Abdominal examination revealed a renal mass. Ultrasound examination of the abdomen revealed a bilateral renal mass.

Questions

1 How would you manage such a child?
2 What is the prognosis?

Answers

1 The most likely diagnosis in a child of this age is a bilateral Wilms' tumour with the most important differential diagnosis being an extensive neuroblastoma. Synchronous bilateral Wilms' tumours account for under 4% of the total cases of Wilms' tumour. Although uncommon it is of paramount importance to establish the diagnosis before starting treatment as treatment options will be significantly influenced. Not all bilateral tumours are diagnosed on preoperative investigations, therefore any patient with a possible Wilms' tumour should be thoroughly investigated to try to detect bilateral disease. These investigations should include an ultrasound examination, an intravenous urogram together with an inferior caval venogram and a CT scan. In spite of these investigations one-third of patients only have the bilaterality of the disease diagnosed

at the time of surgery. Any patient undergoing a nephrectomy for a unilateral Wilms' disease should be explored using a transverse transperitoneal approach. The contralateral kidney should be mobilized and inspected first in order to rule out bilateral disease.

In the patient presented here the ultrasound and intravenous urogram showed the classic findings of Wilms' tumour with calyceal distortion of both kidneys. The inferior caval venogram and ultrasound did not reveal any evidence of tumour within the inferior vena cava. Both tumours were biopsied using a number of passages of a Tru-cut needle biopsy. These biopsies confirmed a favourable histology Wilms' tumour and the patient was started on chemotherapy.

Serial follow up with ultrasound showed good response with tumour regression. A laparotomy was performed at 3 months which confirmed that both tumours had shrunk significantly. It was possible to excise the tumour from each kidney by an appropriate polar heminephrectomy. The child was continued on chemotherapy for a further year. If one of the tumours had not shrunk adequately one would have considered heminephrectomy on the side that had responded and a further biopsy of the non-responsive tumour followed by a course of radiotherapy. The key to surgery of bilateral Wilms' tumours is to be conservative in order to preserve as much functioning renal tissue as possible. Because of the bilaterality of the disease this is obviously not a local defect but is a pan renal abnormality. The prognosis of bilateral Wilms' tumour is in fact good with overall survival at approximately 80%.

Case 7

A 3-year-old girl presented to the outpatient department with a history of persistent wetting during the day and the night. She had never been dry. Physical examination was normal. An ultrasound examination revealed a dilated upper moiety of a duplex right kidney with what appeared to be an enlarged ureter behind the bladder on that side.

Questions

1 What is the differential diagnosis?
2 What further investigations should be done?
3 What role has surgical management in this child?

Answers

1 It is not infrequent for young girls aged 3–4 years to be seen in the outpatient department with a history of wetting. Usually these children have been dry for up to a few months and have then suffered from enuresis and daytime wetting. This is often associated with the symptoms of bladder instability, i.e. urgency, frequency and dampness. This girl's history was not suggestive of bladder instability and the ultrasound findings make the most likely diagnosis that of a duplex right kidney with the upper moiety ureter opening ectopically into the vagina. Girls with a female epispadias who have day- and night-time incontinence because of a failure of normal development of the bladder neck would have normal kidneys on ultrasound. The female epispadias would also be noted on physical examination when the bifid clitoris is seen.

2 This child should be investigated with an intravenous urogram (IVU) which would show a poorly functioning upper moiety of the right kidney with a large ureter displacing the kidney laterally. Sometimes the function is so poor that the upper moiety is not visualized at all on an IVU and neither can the ureter be seen. The diagnosis is then made by the drooping flower appearance of the lower moiety of the kidney together with the displacement caused by the enlarged ectopic ureter pushing the kidney laterally. Some girls with an ectopic ureter have such poor function from the upper pole that not enough urine is produced to lead to incontinence. The few dribbles of dilute urine that are produced remain within the enlarged ectopic ureter and often become infected. These patients then present with either a persistent vaginal discharge or wetting when they are in the upright posture, i.e. during the day. At night, when they are lying down, the ureter gradually fills up with the small amount of urine that is

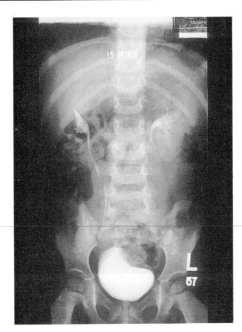

Figure 2 Duplex right kidney

produced by the upper moiety of that kidney and then dribbles out during the day.

3 This child will require surgery to become dry. The three types of operation that are possible are an upper pole heminephrectomy, a ureteropyelostomy or a re-implantation of the ureters into the bladder. The decision as to which type of surgery to perform depends upon the function of the upper moiety of the right kidney. Therefore a DMSA scan should be undertaken to determine the degree of function of the upper moiety. If there is hardly any function then an upper pole heminephrectomy with excision of the ureter as far down as possible from an upper abdominal incision should be undertaken. If there is good function the operative decision lies between a ureteropyelostomy and a double-barrelled re-implantation on that side. If there is a large extrarenal pelvis of the lower

moiety which can be visualized on the IVU a ureteropye-lostomy should be undertaken. If the lower moiety renal pelvis is intrarenal it would make this operation extremely difficult. It is then better to perform a double-barrelled re-implantation of the ureters on that side. These children do well after surgery. It is important always to consider a duplex system with ectopic ureter in girls who are persistently wet or who have a persistent vaginal discharge.

Case 8

A 4-year-old male child presented to casualty with a history of three episodes of haematuria and difficulty in voiding. Clinical examination showed him to be slightly anaemic with a palpable suprapubic mass. Ultrasound showed a mild left hydronephrosis with echogenic material in the bladder. An intravenous urogram confirmed left hydronephrosis with a dilated left ureter and filling defects within the bladder.

Questions

1 What is the most likely diagnosis?
2 How should the child be managed?

Answers

1 The appearances on the intravenous urogram are classic for a bladder rhabomyosarcoma. Rarely, severe cystitis can lead to haematuria and filling defects are present on an intravenous urogram. There is no other differential diagnosis. The diagnosis is made by cystoscopy which reveals a white lobulated mass with polypoid projections within the bladder and biopsy which confirms a rhabdomyosarcoma.
2 Other initial investigations should include a full blood

count, urea and electrolytes and creatinine, urinalysis, intravenous urogram and a chest X-ray. Following confirmation of the diagnosis of bladder rhabdomyosarcoma on histology, further investigations include a CT scan of the pelvis and chest, which showed no evidence of disease elsewhere and a bone marrow aspirate and trephine. These again showed no evidence of disseminated disease. The recommended clinical staging in rhabdomyosarcoma is:

Group 1   Completely resected
Group 2   Microscopic residual disease
Group 3   Gross residual disease
Group 4   Distant metastases

An example of Group 1 disease is that of a paratesticular rhabdomyosarcoma which is completely resected. Following biopsy this patient with Group 3 disease was treated with combination chemotherapy and re-evaluated using ultrasound and biopsy. On follow-up ultrasound at 3 months there was significant tumour shrinkage. This continued for the following 3 months but then appeared to stop. Cystoscopy and biopsy revealed a viable tumour arising from the right lateral wall of the bladder. As there was no further tumour shrinkage treatment options lay between radiotherapy and a cystectomy.

In order to try to preserve the bladder he was given a course of radiotherapy. Unfortunately there was minimal tumour shrinkage at the end of treatment with viable tumour still present. It was felt therefore that we should proceed to a cystectomy. The method of diverting the urine when carrying out a cystectomy for malignant disease in a young child is open to debate. The possibilities include an ileal loop diversion until the child is older, a ureterosigmoidostomy, ureterostomies or a continent diversion. In this patient we elected to perform end ureterostomies as a temporary form of diversion to make sure that there was no obvious recurrent disease within 2 years after cystectomy. In fact the child remained well and as there were problems with fitting a bag on the cutaneous ureterostomies at the age of $6\frac{1}{2}$ a continent urinary diversion using an ileocaecocystoplasty and Mitrofanoff procedure was undertaken. The appendix was brought out in the umbilicus and the child was able to catheterize the caecocystoplasty 4–5 hourly and remain continent and dry. Six years after follow up he remained well. Follow up of his upper tracts was carried out using ultrasound.

Case 9

A boy aged 5 years was seen in the outpatients department with a history of day- and night-time wetting with urgency and frequency. Examination revealed a well child with a palpable bladder which failed to empty after several attempts at micturition. Renal function was normal. The child was otherwise well.

Questions

1 What are the likely causes of the child's symptoms?
2 How can the child be managed?

Answers

1 The differential diagnosis is of an obstructive uropathy of the lower urinary tract or dysfunctional voiding (formerly known as occult neuropathic bladder). Clinical examination apart from the palpable bladder was entirely normal. In particular the legs, spine and lower limb reflexes were normal. There was normal anal tone with a normal anal reflex.
2 This child was investigated with an ultrasound which confirmed a full bladder and mild bilateral hydronephrosis. A cystogram was performed to exclude urethral valves or a urethral diverticulum. The cystogram showed an enlarged thick-walled trabeculated bladder with multiple diverticulae consistent with a neuropathic bladder. The bladder neck appeared normal as was the urethra. With the presence of normal neurology on physical examination a

diagnosis of an occult neuropathic bladder was made. X-rays of the whole vertebral column from the cervical spine to the sacrum were taken to exclude a bony abnormality. A magnetic resonance imaging (MRI) scan of the lumbar sacral spine was also normal.

This patient is at risk from recurrent urinary infections and deteriorating renal function. In order to document bladder function flow rates and ultrasound estimations of residual urine were performed. These showed an interrupted flow rate with a large post void residual volume suggesting detrusor–sphincter–dyssynergia. Because of these abnormalities investigations were pursued with a video cystometrogram (CMG). These patients have normal urethral sensation and it is often better to insert two fine suprapubic catheters into the bladder under general anaesthesia to carry out this investigation rather than trying to introduce a urethral catheter into a nervous child in strange surroundings. The video CMG confirmed a low compliant bladder with high end filling pressure and unstable detrusor contractions. There was failure of relaxation of the external sphincter during the detrusor contraction.

The diagnosis of dysfunctional voiding covers a whole spectrum of abnormalities with the abnormal bladder behaviour either being due to a subsequently diagnosed neuropathy or secondary to a learned behavioural abnormality with detrusor–sphincter–dyssynergia. The family and social history must be investigated. Help, if necessary, from a child psychiatrist should be used if there appears to be a significant psychiatric problem. If it is thought that this is learned detrusor–sphincter–dyssynergia, initial biofeedback should be used to try to get the patient to relax his pelvic floor while attempting to void. Occasionally this will be sufficient to reduce bladder pressure and empty the bladder well enough to avoid further treatment. If it is unsuccessful the child will need to be taught intermittent self catheterization to lower the bladder storage pressure and empty the bladder adequately on a 4-hourly basis. In many patients this is also enough to keep them continent. If compliance is markedly reduced it may occasionally be necessary to augment the bladder, but in dysfunctional voiding this is unusual.

Case 10

A 9-year-old girl presented to the casualty department having been kicked by a horse in the left flank. Examination revealed a well child with a slight tachycardia and obvious left-sided abdominal pain. Examination revealed bruising to the left lower chest consistent with a kick by a horse together with localized tenderness. A urine test confirmed the presence of haematuria.

Question

How would you manage this child?

Answer

This child was not shocked but the likelihood existed that renal injury had occurred in view of the haematuria. A drip should be inserted and blood sent for a full blood count and a group and cross match. Chest X-rays revealed fractures of the lower ribs but no pneumothorax. An abdominal X-ray showed no abnormality. An ultrasound examination should be carried out with particular attention paid to the left kidney and the spleen. The spleen appeared intact but there was evidence of a haematoma around the upper pole of the left kidney. The right kidney appeared normal. In any patient with renal trauma it is important that an intravenous urogram (IVU) is carried out with nephrotomograms if necessary. This will allow classification of the injury to the left kidney, confirm the presence of function or non-function and also confirm the presence of a normal functioning right kidney.

The presence of a non-functioning left kidney indicates the likelihood of vascular disruption of that kidney. Absence of the kidney has been excluded by the ultrasound examination. Non-function of a kidney on an IVU soon after trauma is one of the few indications for renal arteriography in children. There have been rare reports of successful salvage of a kidney following repair of an intimal tear of the renal artery after trauma. The majority of patients with renal trauma will be found to have a functioning kidney with evidence of either a contusion or a laceration to the kidney. Two schools of thought exist regarding treatment of major renal lacerations. These are either surgical or conservative. As in most controversies in surgery, neither side admits to the other's point of view, but in this country the majority of surgeons adopt a conservative approach and only explore a kidney if there is continuing evidence of blood loss in spite of conservative management. If a laparotomy is required it is important that a transperitoneal approach is adopted for two reasons. First, it is important to exclude other intra-abdominal trauma particularly the spleen and liver. Second, it is important before mobilizing the kidney to obtain control of the vascular pedicle and this is best done before opening Gerota's fascia.

The majority of patients treated conservatively will settle down. A DMSA scan should be carried out to define the amount of functioning kidney after recovery from the injury. It is important that patients have their blood pressures monitored regularly after renal trauma as one of the late indications for surgical intervention is hypertension secondary to the renal trauma. Providing the blood pressure remains normal and the DMSA scan shows reasonable function the patient is followed up by the general practitioner.

Case 11

A 2-year-old girl was referred by her general practitioner with a history of recurrent episodes of pyrexia, dysuria and a mid-stream urine (MSU) which grew a significant growth of *Escherichia coli* and more than 100 white cells/mm^3.

Questions

1 How should this girl be investigated?
2 What are the principles of management?

Answers

1 A large number of children referred with a urinary infec-

tion are young girls with lower tract symptoms of dysuria and without a significant pyrexia or episodes of systemic illness. Investigations of these children are often negative. Patients with systemic symptoms may well have significant urinary tract anomalies and should be appropriately investigated. Initial assessment should include a full history with particular reference to the presence of constipation and a voiding history. Many children, in particular girls, are infrequent voiders. Bladder instability with urgency and frequency and incontinence is often associated with positive MSUs. Examination should exclude a palpable bladder and confirm a normal spine and a normal gross neurological examination. The blood pressure must also be taken. In the patient outlined above the history and clinical examination were normal.

Initial investigations should be a plain X-ray of the abdomen and an ultrasound examination of the urinary tract. The plain X-ray will reveal the presence of calculi and whether the lumbar sacral spine is normal. The ultrasound examination revealed a normal left kidney, but a slightly smaller right kidney with a scar of the upper pole and a rather full ureter and pelvis. A likely diagnosis therefore of vesico-ureteric reflux was made. The child was started on prophylactic antibiotics and a micturating cystourethrogram and DMSA scan was performed. The micturating cystourethrogram scan revealed grade 3 reflux on the right side but was otherwise normal. The DMSA scan showed the right kidney to be smaller than the left, contributing 35% of overall renal function and scars present in both the upper and lower poles. The diagnosis of right-sided vesico-ureteric reflux was therefore confirmed with associated chronic pylonephritic damage to the right kidney.

2 The two methods of treatment of this child are either conservative with prophylactic antibiotics, or operative correction of the reflux. There has been little evidence over the years to show that surgical intervention affects the long-term prognosis of patients with vesico-ureteric reflux. This patient was therefore started on prophylactic antibiotics to be taken at night. Attention was also paid to her voiding pattern and the importance of avoiding constipation was reinforced. Prophylaxis in this case should be continued for approximately 2 years with yearly blood

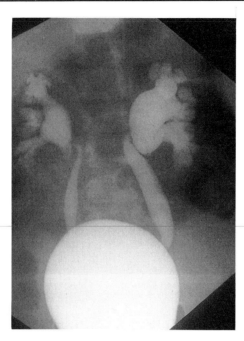

Figure 3 Bilateral vesico-ureteric reflux

pressure checks and MSUs performed if symptoms suggestive of a urinary tract infection occur. After 2 years the DMSA scan and micturating cystogram are repeated. If the reflux has ceased antibiotics are stopped at that time. If reflux persists antibiotics are continued for a further year and then stopped. By the age of six the majority of girls, even if they continue to reflux, stop getting symptomatic urinary infections. If, however, after ceasing the antibiotics symptomatic infections recur again surgery should be considered.

Indications for early surgery are:

1　Failed medical management. This mainly consists of recurrent symptomatic infections in spite of chemo-prophylaxis. Obviously poor compliance of the patient will contribute to this breakthrough infection.
2　Social factors making follow up difficult.
3　Reflux with associated obstruction (rare).

4 Associated bladder pathology in particular large paraureteric diverticulae.

The majority of children do well with conservative treatment. If however surgery is required, two possibilities exist.

1 The Sting procedure is the recently introduced concept of a sub trigonal injection of Teflon or more recently collagen. This has the advantage of not requiring open surgery. It can be carried out as a day case and appears to work well. Long-term follow up however has not yet occurred and therefore one should still be cautious about this type of anti-reflux procedure.

2 Open reimplantation surgery using the trans-trigonal advancement reimplantation (Cohen) technique works well. It is successful in approximately 95% of patients. Complications include significant postoperative obstruction or persisting reflux. Following surgery patients should be reassessed using an ultrasound scan to exclude upper tract dilatation and a cystogram to confirm success of the surgery. Long-term follow up should include yearly blood pressure checks by the general practitioner.

Acute urology

Case 1

A 70-year-old male presented with a history of 48 hours' increasing abdominal pain and desire to void urine but failed to produce any. During the previous 4 days he had frequently voided small volumes of urine with hesitancy. On questioning, he had noted frequency in the day and nocturia (once per night) for several years but had not considered the symptoms troublesome.

On examination the bladder was palpable to the level of the umbilicus. Rectal examination showed a moderately enlarged and clinically benign prostate.

A suprapubic catheter was inserted into the bladder and drained 1800 ml of clear urine. CSU was sterile on culture. Blood urea was 10 mmol/l; Hb 13 g/dl.

Questions

1   What is the pre-existing problem?
2   What further urinary tract investigation is necessary?
3   What management is indicated?

Answers

1   The history and findings in this patient indicated acute on chronic retention of urine and typically he had not been aware of the insidious progress of the condition. The retained volume was far in excess of that expected in simple acute retention (up to 800 ml) with a longer period of failing to void before presentation. Re-examination of the prostate after bladder drainage showed it to be smaller

than was the original impression when a very distended bladder was pushing the gland down on to the examining finger. Chronic retainers often have only modestly enlarged prostates together with a dysfunctional voiding problem and/or detrusor failure.

2   A plain KUB X-ray will show most incidental urinary calculi, calcification in the prostate and larger bone metastases in the case of advanced prostatic carcinoma. Ultrasound will still show signs of upper tract dilatation if present before bladder drainage (an important complication of chronic retention associated with reducing renal function). It may also reveal non-opaque calculi. Further ultrasound information can be obtained from the bladder only if it is full, e.g. the presence of bladder tumours, diverticula and projections of prostate into bladder. Both investigations were negative in this case. In the absence of other symptoms such as haematuria or abnormal signs on ultrasound an IVU rarely adds any further useful information for the management of bladder outlet obstruction and is not routinely necessary.

3   This patient had a transurethral resection of the prostate (TURP) on the next available operating list and was able to void naturally on removal of the postoperative urethral catheter with a residual urine of less than 200 ml, checked by unclamping the suprapubic catheter after voiding prior to its removal. Residual urines below 500 ml are not significant at this stage in cases of chronic retention and will usually reduce if the patient instead of waiting for a desire to void does so by the clock 2 hourly and takes his time to empty the bladder as adequately as possible. Those who fail to void can be sent home with a urethral or suprapubic catheter to return after a month for a trial of voiding which usually succeeds. Those who do not succeed need a further period of drainage by either intermittent self-catheterization if they can cope with it or indwelling catheter if they cannot.

If a suprapubic catheter is used the patient can clamp it intermittently while at home to see if he can void naturally, recording voided volumes if he succeeds and also residual volumes draining into his collecting bag after releasing the clamp. There is no need to disconnect the bag except to change it. Inevitably a few will need to continue with long-term catheters, usually because of lack of mobility, motivation or continuing detrusor failure. These factors need to be taken into account before advising surgery. Antibiotic cover is advisable for all those undergoing surgery for chronic retention and close bacterial monitoring subsequently for those who cannot dispense with catheters shortly after surgery but are expected to do so within a few weeks. Bladder neck stenosis after TURP occasionally occurs if early voiding is not established particularly if a suprapubic rather than a urethral catheter is used for continued drainage.

Some chronic retainers have high tension bladders and are more prone to upper tract dilation with reducing renal function. The bladder is palpably tense as in simple acute retention but painless and the pressure within it is less than a normal voiding pressure. Such patients may produce marked haematuria after decompression of the bladder and have been observed to show hyperaemia and petechiae of the bladder epithelium at this time. Traditional 'slow decompression' by intermittent catheter clamping does not achieve its objective, nor prevent the bleeding. The decompression occurs with the escape of the first few millilitres of urine and even achieving this slowly via a suprapubic 20 ml syringe does not always prevent haematuria. There may be a considerable diuresis after decompression of 'high tension' bladders and a few days' delay for the fluid and electrolyte balance to stabilize before surgery is advisable, particularly for those with renal impairment, using i.v. fluid supplement if necessary.

Chronic retainers without high tension bladders who are still voiding urine and who do not have biochemical evidence of significant renal failure do not need catheter drainage, with its attendant risk of infection, before surgery. Some who have apparent renal impairment and are catheterized, rapidly adjust their biochemistry to normal with a normal fluid intake because they have been drinking very little beforehand in an effort to avoid embarrassing frequency or incontinence. Unfortunately, some patients still present with serious irreversible renal failure and anaemia unaware of their large bladders and the insidious loss of renal function.

Case 2

A 79-year-old male had a one week history of frequency, painful voiding of urine with urgency, hesitancy, poor stream and ultimately inability to void for 6 hours prior to admission. Treatment with a broad spectrum antibiotic had been started by his own doctor. The patient had also had a urinary tract infection treated at home one month previously but had no urinary tract complaints before this. On examination his temperature was 38°C. The bladder was palpable and tender a few centimetres below the umbilicus. Rectal examination showed the prostate to be moderately enlarged with a tense and very tender right lobe which was slightly fluctuant. A suprapubic catheter drained 800 ml of infected urine; the CSU grew *Escherichia coli* sensitive to the antibiotic already started. Blood urea was normal. KUB X-ray and ultrasound of the urinary tract added no further positive information.

Questions

1 What is the diagnosis?
2 What further investigation would you do?
3 What is the management?

Answers

1 The history and signs in this patient are of acute retention of urine with urinary tract infection and the suspicion of an abscess in the right lobe of the prostate.
2 Checking the CSU for sugar, a blood sugar and blood culture were the additional investigations. (They were negative.)
3 The antibiotic treatment was continued and the patient underwent transurethral resection (TUR) drainage of the prostate with the release of a quantity of pus, after which rectal examination on the resectoscope confirmed complete drainage of the right lobe. A postoperative urethral catheter was not used. The patient was able to void naturally after 24 hours and the suprapubic catheter was removed.
    TUR drainage of the prostatic abscess is the immediate

and usually definitive management as in this case. Prostatic abscesses are an occasional cause of acute retention. About half the patients with an abscess will present in this way and others discharge pus spontaneously into the urethra. Diabetics are more prone to prostatic suppuration and the commonest organism cultured is *E. coli* (it used to be *Neisseria gonorrhoeae*). Perhaps, surprisingly, per rectal needle prostatic cytology rarely causes any abscess or urinary tract infection, though tissue core biopsies are more likely to and antibiotic cover is advised for these.

Both cases 1 and 2 had their retention relieved by suprapubic balloon catheters placed with a tear-off strip Nottingham introducer. In the second case, avoidance of the seat of pain and suppuration in draining the bladder was an advantage, although the routine use of suprapubic catheters, as opposed to urethral, for acute retention is debatable. If urethral or prostatic pathology prevents urethral passage with ease then a suprapubic catheter is preferable to the various aids to urethral catheter intro-duction which can be traumatic, although suprapubic catheters also have their complications (haematoma, extra-vasation of urine and perforation of the wrong viscus). Before use of a suprapubic catheter is must be certain that the bladder is distended with urine, using ultrasound if necessary to confirm this, and always obtaining urine via the local anaesthetic needle before catheter introduction 2–3 cm above the symphysis pubis.

Contraindications to the suprapubic route are previous lower abdominal surgery, clot retention and bladder tumours. One advantage of the suprapubic catheter is that trials of voiding are easy and particularly appropriate in acute retention following surgery (other than on the lower abdomen), medication or during the course of another acute illness.

Patients with acute urinary retention are a vulnerable group as a whole with a higher mortality in the first 2 years after surgery than those with 'uncomplicated' bladder outlet obstructive symptoms. Among them will be patients who have serious intercurrent disease and precipitating factors such as cardiopulmonary crises, cerebrovascular incidents and advanced prostatic carcinoma. Selection for surgery needs careful assessment and alternative means of management such as prostatic stenting or continuing indwelling catheter will be more appropriate for the less well.

Case 3

A 21-year-old male was getting out of his car when he experienced sudden pain in the right scrotum. It was constant and severe. He telephoned his general practitioner who told him to get someone to drive him to the local hospital immediately. He vomited on the way. On arrival it was rapidly established that he had no associated lower urinary tract symptoms. Temperature, pulse and BP were normal. (Mid-stream urine later showed no cells and was sterile.) On examination the right scrotum was a little hyperaemic and the right testis highly placed. It was extremely tender and taking the weight off the cord by elevating the testis with one finger did not reduce the pain. The left testis appeared normal in size and orientation. Doppler ultrasound with the probe applied to the lower scrotum showed a pulse deficiency on the affected side. The patient mentioned that 2–3 years previously he had experienced a similar but lesser pain lasting a few hours.

Questions

1 What is the diagnosis?
2 What is the management?
3 What other diagnoses must be considered?

Answers

1 The symptoms and signs indicate testicular torsion.
2 Immediate scrotal exploration is indicated with incision through the tunica vaginalis to examine the testis. In this case the right testis was blue and the cord had twisted through 360°. On untwisting, the testis gradually became pink. It was then apparent that it was lying horizontally with a long mesorchium and high investment of the tunica vaginalis around the spermatic cord. The testis was fixed

with three absorbable sutures passing through the tunica albuginea and the deeper scrotal coverings. The tunica vaginalis was left open. The opposite testis which was explored through a separate scrotal incision, showed similar but lesser anatomical anomalies and was similarly fixed.

In this case the history and signs were of classical and unmistakable torsion of the testis and the history of a previous spontaneously resolving episode of pain is not unusual. Vomiting after torsion is also common. The GP's advice was correct in order to minimize the time between the onset of symptoms and arrival at a place where rapid assessment and exploration could be carried out. It is usually stated that untreated torsion results in the onset of testicular necrosis in 6 hours, but this should not become an allowable time to wait if torsion is suspected, although not all testes twist sufficiently to cause early strangulation. Intravaginal torsion, as opposed to extra-vaginal in neonates, occurs most commonly between the ages of 10 and 19 years. The anatomical abnormalities predisposing are narrow attachment of the tunica vaginalis to the back of the testis, separation of the testis from the epididymis and high investment of the tunica around the spermatic cord. The testis may lie horizontally as a result of this and the abnormality may be noted on the opposite side as a pointer to diagnosis. If seen early it may be possible to demonstrate the gap between the testis and the epididymis but pain and tenderness together with scrotal oedema in the later presentation obscure the signs. The cord may be shorter as a result of torsion retracting the testis to a higher position as in the case described.

3 The important differential diagnoses in this age group are torsion of the appendix testis and acute epididymitis. The former also presents with sudden onset of pain and, in its early stages, a little tender lump at the upper pole of the epididymis can be felt or seen, blue in colour, through the small reactive hydrocele. The testis is not so painful and will usually allow palpation. Acute epididymitis is usually gradual in onset and may be associated with urinary tract infection. Elevation of the testis which is supposed to reduce pain in the case of acute epididymo-orchitis (Prehn's sign) is unreliable. Viral orchitis, which is usually unilateral and not always associated with mumps, rarely occurs

before puberty but must enter the differential diagnosis. Idiopathic scrotal oedema which may affect one or both sides of the scrotum in infants and sometimes extends to adjacent skin, is rapid in onset and while the skin may be tender, the testis can be palpated in the early stages and is not painful.

Confusion can arise between the diagnosis of an irreducible inguinal hernia and torsion of an incompletely descended testis if the scrotum is not carefully palpated to check its contents in the case of a painful groin lump. Moreover, an irreducible inguinal hernia can, by pressure on the cord vessels, compromise the blood supply of a normally placed testis in young children.

On paper, differentiation between all these conditions is simpler than in practice. Use of the Doppler ultrasound probe applied to the lower scrotum may show a diminished pulse in torsion but reactive hyperaemia on the affected side in torsion may diminish the difference, in which case pressure with a finger on the cord of the affected side may make little difference to the audible pulse compared with the same procedure on the unaffected side. Isotope scanning to display presence or absence of testicular perfusion has been shown to be a much more accurate investigation, but not generally recommended nor available at short notice. Colour Doppler has the potential to resolve the question of testicular perfusion and it remains to be seen if it finds a place alongside clinical assessment.

When all is said and done, if there is doubt, exploration should be carried out after permission has been granted to remove the testis if it is dead and to fix the opposite side. In any case, torsion of the appendix testis is relieved more quickly by excising it rather than treating with analgesics and then having second thoughts about the diagnosis later. Exploration in a doubtful case of epididymo-orchitis is less harmful than delay in diagnosis of a torsion (resulting in testicular loss).

The testis must be clearly dead to indicate removal; necrotic or infarcted with no restoration of circulation after untwisting, so many doubtful testes are left in situ and undergo subsequent atrophy. The matter of whether the dying testis induces an autoimmune process which will interfere with the products of the live one is as yet not wholly resolved. Finally, a testicular prosthesis, if required, is placed at a later date.

Case 4

A 38-year-old male was referred to outpatients with a 3-month history of pain and a palpable swelling in the left scrotum. During this time he had had three different antibiotics prescribed. Each treatment was associated with a transient reduction in symptoms and signs. There were no associated urinary tract symptoms, no previous history of them and no recollection of any serious illness. He and his wife had been attending a sub-fertility clinic for some years. Oligospermia had been noted.

On examination there was a tender firm swelling, about 2 cm across, in the upper pole of the left epididymis, the right side felt normal. A month's course of trimethoprim was prescribed, a mid-stream urine (MSU) taken and an ultrasound of the scrotal contents arranged. The patient was seen again in 2 weeks: the MSU had shown an excess of white cells but was sterile on culture, and the ultrasound showed enlargement of the upper pole of the left epididymis which contained a 1 cm cavity consistent with an abscess, the testis appeared normal. Exploration under anaesthesia showed inflammation of the epididymis with a secondary lax hydrocele. A thick-walled abscess in the upper pole was drained, culture was sterile and in the meantime a further MSU showed persistent white cells but no growth on culture.

Questions

1 What underlying cause for these findings is suspected?
2 What investigations should be carried out?

Answers

1 Tuberculosis should have been suspected on the initial findings, i.e. oligospermia, unresolving epididymitis on antibiotic treatment and the finding of sterile pyuria persisting long after repeated antibiotic treatment. Unfortunately a Ziehl-Neelsen stain of the epididymal pus for mycobacteria was not done, neither was histology of the abscess wall which might have shown the characteristics of TB.

2 Further evidence of tuberculous infection should be sought. Three early morning specimens of the urine were sent for TB culture, chest X-ray was normal, KUB X-ray showed a little calcification at the upper pole of the left kidney and subsequent intravenous urogram (IVU) revealed a calyceal stricture in association with this. The rest of the urinary tract was normal. Finally a Mantoux test was strongly positive and during the course of these investigations, although the scrotal incision healed, the inflammation failed to show any signs of resolution. Anti-tuberculous therapy was started under the supervision of an infectious diseases specialist and the urine cultures eventually returned positive for tuberculosis, sensitive to the prescribed chemotherapy. The patient's wife was investigated and found to have no evidence of tuberculosis, genital or otherwise. (It is unusual for TB to be transmitted via the genital tract.) The patient's epididymal lesion resolved, urine microscopy became normal and a further IVU at 12 months showed the calyceal stricture had dilated a little. The sperm counts were below normal with poor motility and sperm antibodies were detected in the peripheral blood.

The incidence of tuberculous epididymitis has been declining in most western countries and while it is occasionally seen in older people, sometimes presenting with secondary infection such as *Escherichia coli*, sporadic cases occur in younger, sexually active men who are the usual sufferers in countries where the disease is common. Although there may be a history of TB or association with upper urinary tract disease (not usually cystitis or prostatitis), epididymitis may be the only manifestation of the infection which is blood borne, affecting the upper pole of the epididymis initially. Involvement of the lower pole, the vas deferens (beading) and the development of a posterior scrotal sinus occurs in more advanced cases but testicular involvement, which may be indistinguishable on examination from a tumour, is not common. The presentation in western countries is usually early, with a low-grade epididymitis, occasionally following an acute episode, which persists and fails to respond to antibiotic treatment. If after one month's antibiotic treatment there is no response, evidence of TB elsewhere should be sought as described in this patient. Ultrasound may be helpful in differentiating between a testicular and epididymal mass and will identify a small epididymal abscess which requires drainage. A strongly positive Mantoux test is likely to indicate active tuberculosis rather than past infection or BCG conversion but the response can be modified by steroid therapy and other immunodeficient states as well as chronic illness. Anti-TB therapy is therefore advocated by some for unresponsive epididymitis without positive confirmation of the diagnosis and if the therapy fails then exploration is indicated because of the possibility of testicular tumour.

Nowadays, epididymal pain and congestion following vasectomy (sometimes years after) may be confused with unresolving epididymitis. Epididymectomy and excision of the vas up to the vasectomy site may be indicated for this condition.

Case 5

A 72-year-old man with chronic obstructive airway disease was admitted 2 days after the onset of severe, constant right loin pain, fever and anuria. He had vomited three times on the day of admission.

On examination, he appeared dehydrated, slightly cyanosed, temperature 38.5°C, pulse 90, BP 160/80, respiratory rate 30 per minute with a productive cough and yellow sputum. Coughing caused pain in the right lower chest and also aggravated the right loin pain. There were otherwise no grossly abnormal clinical signs in the chest, the right loin was tender. The urinary bladder was not palpable. A chest X-ray showed slightly increased opacity over the right lung but no localized changes. Blood urea was 23 mmol/l, creatinine 722 mmol/l, sodium 130 mmol/l, potassium 5 mmol/l, HCO_3 17.3, Hb 13 g/dl. KUB X-ray showed an excess of gas throughout the colon and a possible right ureteric calculus adjacent to the body of L3.

Ultrasound showed a larger than normal right kidney with a small renal pelvis and the left kidney could not be detected. An intravenous urogram (IVU) showed a faint nephrogram on the right with no outline of either the renal pelvis or ureter. There was no function on the left side. A urethral catheter was passed, draining a few millilitres of infected urine which was sent for culture. Sputum and blood were also sent for culture after a peripheral blood white cell count of $24\,000 \times 10^9/l$ was noted. Intramuscular amoxycillin was started.

Questions

1 How should the investigation proceed?
2 What is the management?

Answers

1 Clinical uncertainty was expressed in the admission notes as to whether this patient was suffering primarily from a pulmonary or renal problem, although investigation soon confirmed anuria and a solitary obstructed kidney, probably by a calculus, though this was not clear on a plain X-ray partially obscured by faecal and gas shadowing. The IVU could not be expected to produce very informative films in the presence of anuria with a high serum creatinine, but did outline one functioning kidney. The raised temperature and white count together with the other constitutional signs were consistent with septicaemia secondary to pyonephrosis.

2 The immediate need was to secure drainage of the kidney and ultrasound guided percutaneous nephrostomy under local anaesthesia in this sick man was the procedure of choice on the initial ultrasound findings. The radiologist, however, felt that he could not successfully access the small pelvi-calyceal system (acute obstruction does not produce much distension of the pelvi-calyceal system particularly if it is initially small or intra-renal). The patient was therefore taken to an operating theatre equipped with a C-arm image intensifier and under general anaesthesia cystoscopy showed a little pus exuding from a solitary right ureteric orifice, the left was absent, confirming the ultrasound diagnosis of a solitary right kidney.

The presence of a suspected calculus was confirmed as a blunt-ended stent was passed up the ureter and arrested as it reached the 1 cm diameter opacity but would not pass it. The stent was therefore removed and in its place a floppy-ended guidewire was introduced which passed the calculus and allowed the stent to be guided up to the kidney releasing a gush of murky urine into the bladder as the wire was withdrawn.

Stents can displace calculi in the uppermost part of the ureter back into the renal pelvis but the distance of the stone from the renal pelvis in this case was not clear. Had the procedure failed, then open surgery would have been carried out to remove the stone and secure drainage. In the event, urinary excretion of 60 ml an hour was immediately established and increased during the next few hours with appropriate i.v. fluid replacement governed by central venous pressure measurements and monitoring the plasma urea and electrolyte levels. With recovery in renal performance the patient's biochemical state improved over the next week by which time the blood urea was 15.4 mmol/l and creatinine 250 mmol/l. Blood and urine cultures isolated *E. coli* sensitive to the amoxycillin first prescribed. There is a tendency to use more recently introduced broad spectrum antibiotics in cases of septicaemia originating from the urinary tract, but nephro-toxicity must be taken into account and blood levels monitored. Subsequent extracorporeal shock wave lithotripsy on this patient was successful and the stent later removed at 3 months, rather a long time in a stone former, in whom there is a risk of stent encrustation, but KUB X-rays showed the stent to be clean in this case.

Ideally, such a patient is much better managed from the outset in a renal unit where there is a high level of expertise available for percutaneous renal access as well as the necessary experience to manage renal failure before and after the return of renal function.

Case 6

A 69-year-old woman was admitted to hospital with a history of 24 hours' left loin pain. She had suffered a similar pain for 2 days the week previously and 2 months before this, transient pain in the right loin. She was not aware of passing any calculi and had no lower urinary tract symptoms. Ten years previously she had undergone vaginal surgery for repair of a prolapse. She was afebrile, BP 130/90. Apart from tenderness in the left loin there were no abnormal signs on examination of the abdomen. Mid-stream urine showed no cells and was sterile on culture. A KUB X-ray showed no opacities in the line of the urinary tract and the next day an intravenous urogram (IVU) showed a normal right kidney and ureter, but, on the left side excretion was delayed showing a faint outline of the upper urinary tract to the level of lumbar vertebra 4 where there appeared to be a tapering obstruction in the ureter. The distal ureter was not adequately displayed at this examination.

Questions

1 How would you proceed with investigation and management?
2 How would you next proceed on the findings given?

Answers

1 A tapering stricture of the ureter in the absence of any other primary signs in the kidney and a normal urine indicates a search for a cause of external ureteric compression such as retro-peritoneal malignancy, irradiation, aortic pathology or medication induced fibrosis. Further questioning and examination of the patient failed to reveal any pointers to these possible causes and routine blood examinations both haematological and biochemical, were normal. Cystoscopy and gynaecological examination under anaesthesia were unremarkable. A catheter was introduced into the left ureter with ease and retrograde ureterography in the theatre showed the stricture to be about 5 cm in length. A double pig-tail stent was similarly introduced with ease and a CT scan booked to examine the posterior abdominal wall. There was a delay of some weeks before CT was achieved and when it was the patient had begun to experience right loin pain and a right hydronephrosis was observed with a hydro-ureter down to the level of the aortic bifurcation. Around the aorta and inferior vena cava there was a soft tissue mass which was not large but was poorly defined, suggestive of retroperitoneal fibrosis. A double pig-tail stent was therefore placed in the right

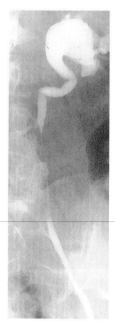

Figure 4 Retrograde left ureteropyelography showing partial obstruction associated with narrow ureteric segment tapered at both ends

ureter. At laparotomy 4 weeks later the retroperitoneal fat around the aortic bifurcation and just above was thickened and inflamed. Petechiae arose on the peritoneum after gentle palpation and the changes were more in evidence on the left side covering the ureter from view whereas on the right side the ureter appeared free from encroachment. The aorta showed a little atheroma on palpation but was of a normal diameter.

2   It was decided to mobilize the left ureter only. Tissue from the affected retroperitoneal fat was sent for frozen section histology, the result was equivocal with some suspicion of malignancy so further tissue was sent for later paraffin sections. The ureter mobilized easily and was enclosed in a flap of peritoneum raised from the left abdomen. Subsequent histology of the retroperitoneal biopsy showed inflammatory changes only.

The left and right stents were removed at 2 and 4 months respectively after surgery and 8 months after surgery an IVU showed normal ureters and no obstruction on either side.

There is recent evidence that many cases of 'idiopathic' retroperitoneal fibrosis represent a peri-aortitis which in its grossest form is associated with an inflammatory abdominal aortic aneurysm but may be associated with a normal diameter slightly atheromatous aorta. Moreover, the condition seems to be self-limiting in some cases and steroid treatment can also have a place in bringing about a resolution. In some, however, prolonged stenting and the use of steroids does not resolve the problem and ureterolysis in these cases is therefore indicated.

The time intervals in this case between investigation and surgical intervention saw the retro-peritoneal changes developing and resolving to some extent simply with the passage of time and the patient remained symptom free 18 months later. Ultrasound in follow up will show if there is any recurrence of hydronephrosis. The use of stents allows time to elapse and resolution to occur with or without the use of steroids before it is necessary to contemplate surgery.

In retrospect, a trial of steroids with the stents might have solved the problem for this patient. In the event, surgery took the credit for relieving obstruction of the left ureter and no doubt would have done so for the right if bilateral ureterolysis had been undertaken at the time.

Case 7

A 48-year-old healthy patient had undergone abdominal hysterectomy with conservation of the ovaries for fibroids and dysmenorrhoea. The operation was apparently straight-forward. A peroperative urethral catheter was removed 2 days after surgery after which she voided urine naturally but had an *Escherichia coli* urinary tract infection treated with trimethoprim. It was also noted that she had a vaginal discharge for 3 days after operation. At 10 days, after returning home, she began to leak clear fluid vaginally, although continuing to void a variable amount of urine, usually small volumes. Some weeks elapsed before her return to hospital when vaginal examination showed a small defect in the closed vaginal vault. A urethral catheter was inserted into the bladder and methylene blue dye introduced through it duly stained the deeply placed end of a vaginal tampon. The catheter was left in the bladder and the clear vaginal leakage reduced to a small volume.

Questions

1 What is the diagnosis?
2 How should investigation proceed?
3 What is the management?

Answers

1 The history is that of a urinary fistula communicating with the vaginal vault from a ureter or the bladder. In the case of a ureteric leak, urine from the opposite upper tract would continue to be voided naturally from the bladder. Natural voiding would also continue in the case of a small vesico-vaginal fistula. Delay in the onset of symptoms after surgery is common and leakage may also be intermittent in the case of a small fistula. The dye test indicated a vesico-vaginal communication assuming that there was no vesico-ureteric reflux, but the test can be messy and inconclusive if dye leaks down the urethra around the catheter and stains the superficially placed part of the tampon.
2 A mid-stream urine and high vaginal swab are taken for culture and any infection treated. An intravenous urogram (IVU) is carried out in the absence of a bladder catheter, paying particular attention to the distal ureters for any sign of obstruction or extravasation as well as to the bladder and vagina, using oblique views as necessary. IVU in this instance showed a normal upper urinary tract and clearly demonstrated a fistula from the lower part of the back of the bladder into the vagina. The diagnosis was therefore confirmed, although in some cases further radiological investigations may be necessary at the next stage which is examination under anaesthetic and cystoscopy. This can be

a separate investigation or a preliminary to fistula repair depending on the complexity of findings and the state of the viscera involved. Repair should not be attempted before any pelvic inflammatory changes or haematoma have resolved and, in the case of recent irradiation, time must elapse to judge its effects on the primary pathology and allow secondary effects on adjacent tissue to stabilize before deciding on its repair (or occasionally urinary diversion).

3   Cystoscopy in the case described showed a small defect in the midline just above the trigone. Examination under anaesthesia showed no other pelvic pathology so repair proceeded immediately. Some post-hysterectomy fistulae are very small and difficult to see at cystoscopy but cannot be expected to heal with a further period of bladder drainage if time has elapsed between the initial symptoms of leakage and re-catheterization of the bladder. Although some fistulae diagnosed early after hysterectomy have been reported to have healed with continued catheterization, once the track is epithelialized, it remains patent like a pierced earlobe.

Vesico-vaginal defects vary considerably in size and complexity depending on the cause and underlying pathology. Obstructed labour with pressure necrosis between the bladder and vaginal wall is well documented, for instance, in southern Africa. Irradiation of locally invasive cervical cancer produces some of the most difficult fistulae to treat. Post-hysterectomy urinary fistulae are more likely to occur after difficult surgery and postoperative infection or in association with anaemia, steroid treatment, diabetes or pelvic irradiation, but may follow apparently straightforward and uncomplicated surgery as in the case described. It is in this latter group where immediate re-catheterization of the bladder at the first sign of urinary leakage might secure healing of a small fistula.

Operative repair requires complete excision of the fistula which involves opening the bladder and the vagina and carefully dissecting the two apart before closure is achieved with absorbable sutures. At operation the patient is placed in a position to give access to the vagina as well as the abdomen. Depending on the size of the fistula and the degree of adjacent tissue fibrosis, it may be necessary to enter the plane between the vagina and the bladder from below and complete the dissection from above. Adequate bladder and ureteric mobilization, if necessary, avoids repair under tension as does an oblique incision in the bladder rather than a vertical one down to the fistula. In the case described an abdominal approach only was made and relatively little dissection required. The bladder is drained with a catheter for 7 days after repair and a suprapubic one has the advantage of a simple trial of voiding before removal avoiding the disappointment of urethral re-catheterization in the case of early voiding failure.

Case 8

A 19-year-old male was brought to hospital after receiving a sharp blow in the right loin on colliding with another player during a football match. He was pale, pulse 86 and BP 90/55 with persistent loin pain. Right loin and abdominal tenderness with guarding was noted. Intravenous access was gained, blood taken for haemoglobin, haematocrit, blood grouping with cross match of 4 units and an i.v. drip started. Chest X-ray was normal, an abdominal film showed increased opacity on the right side with loss of psoas outline and no discernible renal shadow. Within half and hour, and less than 500 ml of i.v. fluid the pulse rate fell and BP rose to 140/80.

Questions

1 What are the likely differential diagnoses?
2 How would you proceed to investigate?
3 What are the management options?

Answers

1 Renal and/or liver trauma with limited blood loss are suspected on the history and findings so far. Immediate ultrasound and intravenous urogram (IVU) are required.
2 Ultrasound showed a large haematoma around the right

renal upper pole and a small collection of fluid around the lower pole. The left kidney, spleen and liver appeared normal.

IVU showed prompt bilateral contrast excretion with a normal left upper tract. All parts of the right kidney functioned but the lower pole was a little separated from the rest with extravasation around it. The ureter was not seen, even on a delayed film and filling defects (probably clots) were seen in the renal pelvis. The patient produced blood-stained urine in X-ray. Observations remained stable.

3   At this stage it was decided to manage conservatively with continued observation including ultrasound monitoring of intra-abdominal signs daily. Antibiotic cover was started. Although the ureter was not seen on X-ray, injury to it was most unlikely with this history and obstruction with clot was suspected. Ureteric injuries, apart from intraoperative causes, are uncommon. They are associated with penetrating wounds (gunshot rather than stabbing) and IVU usually shows them.

In this case, ultrasound showed an increasing urinoma over 24 hours so drainage was required. A percutaneous nephrostomy attempt successfully placed a drain in the urinoma but failed to access the renal collecting system which would have allowed an attempt to intubate and stent the ureter to establish internal drainage. Further X-rays with contrast introduced through the drain outlined the urinoma and entered the renal collecting system, but, as on the IVU, failed to enter the ureter. It was therefore decided on the next day to carry out cystoscopy and retrograde ureterography under general anaesthesia. Ureterography showed the ureter to be uninjured and a double pig-tail stent was placed in it to secure internal drainage, confirmed by further X-ray with contrast through the external drain. There was neither pain nor further urinoma collection when the drain was clamped so it was removed the day after the stent was placed.

Antibiotic cover instituted before the percutaneous drain insertion was continued for 5 days.

In retrospect, the stent may not have been required since normal ureteric drainage could have been re-established as the obstructing clots lysed, but could be justified on the grounds that early removal of the percutaneous drain would reduce access for infection.

The patient was discharged one week after the injury and the stent removed after 2 months. At 3 months an IVU showed an almost normal right kidney. Blood pressure remained normal and should be checked again at intervals for 4 years on the grounds that hypertension may result from renal damage.

The diagnosis of renal injury alone was confirmed in this case although associated liver and splenic injuries are common and these can also be managed conservatively if signs indicate early cessation of haemorrhage. Ultrasound is a most helpful diagnostic and monitoring investigation for all such blunt injuries bearing in mind the development of urinoma, sepsis and secondary haemorrhage which blunt renal truma can produce. Immediate IVU is essential if renal injury is suspected in order to define the extent of the injury and confirm contralateral function. This investigation is part of the early assessment of abdominal injury in some trauma centres. The association with other injuries can mask renal damage and abnormal kidneys are more prone to injury, even with apparently minor trauma. Macroscopic haematuria is not always a feature of renal injury and some produce only microscopic amounts of blood in the urine or none at all, as in the case of some predicle injuries which completely devitalize the kidney, so even microscopic haematuria needs full investigation. The renal vessels are the only firm anchorage point for the kidney and sudden deceleration injuries can damage the vessel walls resulting in thrombosis or varying degrees of avulsion.

Most blunt renal injuries can be treated wholly conservatively with occasional percutaneous nephrostomy/ drainage for urinomas which do not resolve rapidly. Indications for exploration in blunt trauma are continuing haemorrhage and partial or complete non-function of the kidney on IVU, the latter indicating severe disruption or pedicle injury. The approach should be anterior, through the abdomen, in order to gain rapid access to and control of the renal vessels to avoid further serious haemorrhage as the haematoma is explored. In this way the chances of salvaging part or whole of the kidney are enhanced.

Complete IVU non-function in the absence of any other immediate indication for surgery, as is the case in some pedicle injuries, calls for renal arteriography. However, if there is to be an expectation of renal salvage by restoring perfusion before warm ischaemic time is exceeded, the investigation must be achieved without delay and with the operating theatre ready, otherwise any surgery is then to remove the dead organ in order to avoid subsequent infection or secondary haemorrhage.

In practice, the results of pedicle reconstruction are disappointing and the maximum permissible warm ischaemic time is often exceeded before surgery is possible. Some kidneys which have undergone 'auto-nephrectomy' in the stable patient have been managed conservatively or gone undiagnosed until later for want of early investigation.

Penetrating injuries of the kidney associated with gunshot wounds invariably involve other organs and all require surgical exploration. Exploration is also the conventional management of stab wounds, since although some may cause no more damage than uncomplicated percutaneous renal operation, associated visceral and vascular injuries are common and may not be apparent on initial investigation. During recent years however, in some centres where stab injuries are common, many have been treated conservatively in the absence of severe haemorrhage or immediate signs of additional organ involvement. If this policy is adopted very close observation and awareness of complications is necessary for conservatively managed patients and the commonest complication, which is secondary haemorrhage, may not occur until some weeks after the injury. Criteria for a decision not to operate are imprecise at present and it remains to be seen whether improved imaging techniques such as contrast CT will make selection and management simpler and safer.

The decision to explore in cases of major blunt or penetrating injuries involving the kidney has often been taken because of the other injuries and the urologist might be invited to the operating theatre without the help of a preoperative IVU. In these cases the limiting factors for survival of the patient rest with the associated injuries, not with the kidney. It is not too late however, to obtain an IVU on the operating table.

Case 9

A 19-year-old male was brought to the accident and emergency department after the car in which he was travelling collided with a tree. He had suffered injuries to the head, pelvis and left femur and was admitted by the orthopaedic service. The head injury was not serious and X-rays confirmed the fracture of the femoral shaft and of the right pelvis with upward and inward displacement of the acetabulum. During the course of assessment it was noted that a small amount of blood with a tail of clot had leaked from the external urinary meatus. After resuscitation, when the patient had stabilized, it was decided that the femur required internal fixation but before this the urologist was called. Examination showed that the lower abdomen was rather tense and the bladder could not be palpated with certainty. The external genitalia were normal, although there was some fullness of the perineum. Rectal examination was unsatisfactory (the patient had traction splints applied to each lower limb). The patient was equivocal about a desire to void urine and could not manage to. The urologist arranged further investigation.

Questions

1 What sequence of investigations were indicated?
2 What is the management on the findings described?

Answers

1 Blood at the external urinary meatus and a displaced fracture of the pelvis, or either of these findings alone after trauma, indicate the need for imaging of the urinary tract, firstly with intravenous urography (IVU). IVU in this case showed a normal upper tract but the bladder, which was intact, was located higher than usual in the pelvis. Retrograde urethrography was therefore carried out and showed extravasation of contrast from the region of the membraneous urethra. The combination of radiological signs indicated urethral disruption and displacement of the bladder which occurs when the prostate comes adrift from

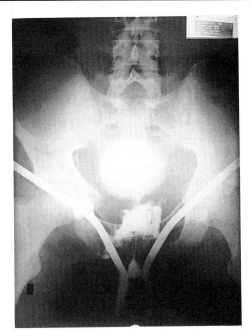

Figure 5 IVU and urethrogram showing displaced bladder and extravasation from urethral rupture

its pelvic attachments, allowing both it and the bladder to be displaced upwards and backwards by the pelvic haematoma (associated with the fracture), thus creating a gap between the two parts of the injured urethra. Although it may be possible to detect prostatic displacement on rectal examination this is not always easy in such an injured patient.

Only about one in ten people with pelvic fractures sustain a urethral injury and few of these are complete ruptures with displacement. Experience in diagnosis and dealing with the serious posterior urethral injury is therefore spread thinly with varied opinion as to the practicalities of management, although the aim, which is universally accepted, is to minimize the subsequently expected stricture. The strictures most difficult to treat are those resulting from wide separation of the urethral ends when later it may be impossible to close the gap by perineal anastomotic repair because of fibrosis causing lack of mobility and elasticity of the bulbomembranous urethra. Urethral re-alignment with reduction in the gap shortly after injury should therefore be achieved in these cases by an experienced urologist, but patients with serious pelvic fractures may have multiple injuries which take priority over the urethral injury.

2 In the case of a displaced pelvic fracture IVU should be incorporated into the assessment as early as possible to see if the bladder is displaced or ruptured. Urethrography should follow if the bladder is displaced or the patient cannot void urine. Ultrasound is also useful in demonstrating whether the bladder is full or empty (if empty is it ruptured or is the patient not secreting urine yet?). If urethral rupture and obvious displacement of the bladder are seen, retropubic exploration is indicated. Clot is evacuated from the retropubic space and the bladder opened. A soft inert self-retaining balloon catheter can now be passed through the anterior urethra across the gap to be guided through the posterior urethra into the bladder. The urethra has now been re-aligned and the procedure is completed leaving an additional suprapubic catheter in the bladder and a suction drain to the retropubic space. This technique was used in the case described and was also sufficient to close the gap between the urethral ends. At the same time, the femoral fracture was internally splinted. Few urologists attempt to secure approximation of the urethral ends by primary urethral repair over the re-alignment catheter. If the gap persists after re-alignment the prostate can be anchored as near as possible to its normal position by two sutures (to be removed later) passing up from the perineal skin through the prostate capsule and out again to be tied over the perineal skin, but this is not easy to achieve. Catheter traction has also been recommended, but if well maintained on a balloon catheter, it risks pressure necrosis around the bladder neck resulting in another stricture.

The timing of intervention depends on the threat to the patient from other injuries. It is best delayed until this is assessed and the patient is stable. It should also coincide with any orthopaedic procedure to fix vertically displaced pelvic fractures and a delay of a few days may reduce the amount of bleeding after clot evacuation, but after 10 days organizing blood clot and fibrosis will make the urethral approximation much more difficult. During the interval between injury and surgery a percutaneous suprapubic catheter, introduced as soon as the bladder is full, drains the urine.

Suprapubic catheterization (which is advocated by some for the expectant management of all bulbomembranous injuries), is used as the sole treatment for complete or partial posterior urethral ruptures where the patient is unable to void urine but does not have a displaced bladder with wide distraction of the urethral ends. Avoidance of urethral catheterization in partial rupture is on the grounds that it may, by trauma or infection, increase the urethral damage. The use of a urethral catheter as a diagnostic aid remains controversial. Some advocate a gentle aseptic trial of urethral catheterization, proceeding to suprapubic catheterization if this fails. The alternative is to leave the urethra uncatheterized and to make the diagnosis by contrast radiography placing the suprapubic catheter as soon as possible to drain and monitor urine output. Whatever method has been used in initial management, urethrography in all cases at 3 weeks with contrast introduced through the suprapubic catheter or the slowly withdrawn urethral catheter will demonstrate whether extravasation persists. If it does, both the re-alignment catheter if any, and the suprapubic should be left for further urethrography in 2 weeks. When healing is demonstrated a trial of voiding can be carried out by clamping the suprapubic catheter. In most cases any stricture can be dealt with by urethrotomy or dilatation at a later date. In the case described, urethrography at 3 weeks showed no extravasation. The patient voided well and only after 10 months did he complain of reduced voiding stream. The bulbar stricture seen at urethroscopy was about 6 French gauge in size and was incised with a direct vision urethrotome. Flow rates remained satisfactory at 6 months.

Stones disease

Case 1

A 34-year-old man presented with the sudden onset of severe pain in the left loin. The pain started at 5.30 a.m. initially localized to the loin but then radiated down into the left iliac fossa and left testicle within the first hour. His general practitioner was called and the patient was given an injection of pethidine 100 mg intramuscularly stat. This settled the pain but 12 hours later a further bout of severe pain occurred, associated with vomiting. The general practitioner referred the patient to hospital.

On admission the patient was in obvious pain and found it difficult to lie still. He was apyrexic with a pulse rate of 72 per minute. Abdominal palpation revealed tenderness in the left loin and in the left iliac fossa. On routine testing of the urine, blood was noted to be present.

A plain X-ray of the urinary tract (KUB) was performed and this showed a small opacity in the true pelvis lying just below the left sacroiliac joint, in line between the joint and the ischial spine. The patient was given a diclofenac suppository and the pain settled overnight. The following morning an intravenous urogram (IVU) was performed (Figure 6). The plain film showed that the opacity had moved to the level of the ischial spine. The right kidney and ureter appeared normal but there was delayed excretion of contrast on the left side. The 45-minute film revealed dilute contrast in a hydronephrotic kidney; a further film was taken 2 hours later and this showed contrast in a slightly distended ureter down to the level of the opacity in the pelvis. The size of the calculus was about 3 mm in diameter. The patient was free of pain for 24 hours so he was discharged home with a supply of diclofenac 50 mg to be taken if necessary and instructions to pass urine into a urine

51

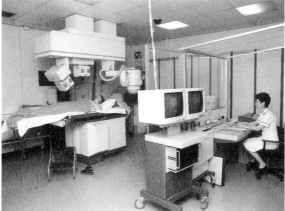

Figure 6 The Siemens Lithostar

bottle so he could retrieve the stone if possible. In fact he passed the small calculus spontaneously after a further short bout of colic. Analysis of the stone revealed calcium oxalate and phosphate. The patient was screened for hypercalcaemia and hypercalciuria.

Questions

1 What complications may follow an IV urogram?
2 Is there any alternative to the IV urogram?
3 What is the plan of management of a stone in the lower third of the ureter?
4 If the attacks of renal colic continue at frequent intervals what further action may be taken?

Answers

1 Adverse reactions to the contrast medium occur in about 5% of people and in 70% of cases they arise within 5 minutes of the intravenous injection. Minor reactions such as a transient hot flush are common; more serious ones associated with nausea and vomiting occur more

commonly with ionic than with non-ionic media. Vaso-vagal attacks are more common with the non-ionic preparations. Reactions consist either of an acute or a delayed acute hypersensitivity manifesting reactions such as urticaria, mild hypotension, headache, bronchospasm or cardio-vascular problems. Acute cardiovascular and/or respiratory collapse may occur as an anaphylactic reaction on rare occasions and appropriate drugs for treating these, including adrenaline, cortisone and antihistamine preparations should always be readily available. Death has been recorded but it is estimated to be a chance of about 1 in 30–40 000 cases. The non-ionic preparations which are now available as radiographic contrast media are expensive but they have reduced the risk of serious reactions. The atopic patient who is at risk may benefit from a pretreatment dose of steroid or antihistamine.

2   Ultrasonography and radionuclide imaging have been proposed as alternatives to the IV urogram. It has been suggested that ultrasonic scanning might replace the urogram but this depends on the stone being situated in a position which is amenable to ultrasonic imaging and the presence of obstruction. Similarly the DTPA scan can be used to triage those patients with ureteric obstruction but not all patients with ureteric stones have obstruction. Urography still remains the linch pin in the evaluation of patients with renal colic but both ultrasound and radionuclide imaging have a place in the follow up of these patients and they can be used as the primary investigation in patients who have experienced a previous hypersensitivity reaction to contrast medium.

3   The larger the stone the less likely it is to pass spontaneously. A stone of less than 4 mm in diameter has about a 90% chance of passing spontaneously if situated in the lower half of the ureter and about an 80% chance in the upper ureter.

Stones 4–6 mm in diameter have about a 50% chance of passing spontaneously if situated in the ureter and those larger than 6 mm have less than a 5% chance if placed in the upper half of the ureter and about a 20% chance in the lower ureter.

The initial management of a small stone in the lower ureter is thus conservative. Patients should normally be treated with analgesics and encouraged to move around freely. If the patient is free of pain for 24 hours he may be allowed home and given diclofenac 50 mg to take orally when necessary. He should be given instructions to report back to the hospital if he has further attacks of pain. Arrangements should be made to see him again within 2 weeks for a further plain X-ray (KUB) to assess whether the stone has advanced. The patient should be asked to retrieve the stone if it is passed so that it can be sent for chemical analysis.

4   A stone in the lower ureter may be treated by extra-corporeal shock wave lithotripsy (ESWL) or extracted via a ureteroscope. ESWL can be performed if the stone is large enough to be localized radiologically. Some lithotripters which have this facility such as the Dornier MPL 9000 or the Siemens Lithostar, can be used for stones in the lower half of the ureter. Those lithotripters which employ ultrasound localization can only be used for larger calculi in the upper ureter or lower ureter adjacent to the bladder. A stone 3 mm in diameter could be difficult to localize on the lithotripter and thus endoscopic extraction would normally be more appropriate.

Before embarking on the extraction of ureteric stones it is prudent to check that radiological facilities are available in the theatre during the procedure. It is not possible to predict whether the operation will take a matter of minutes or much longer and it may be important to screen the ureter or take an X-ray film if difficulties are encountered. The patient should be placed on the operating table without too much hip flexion so that the ureter is kept as straight as possible. Finally choose a cystoscope of 23 or 25 FG which will allow the passage of ureteric dilators at least up to size 12 FG.

The narrowest portion of the ureter is the intramural part hence calculi can become impacted at this point. If this should occur cystoscopic examination of the bladder normally reveals a swollen oedematous ureteric orifice with a bulge above this indicating the site of the stone. Caution is necessary in this situation. It can be difficult to pass a guide wire or any type of dilator and relatively easy to end up with an even more oedematous and bruised ureteric orifice. A diathermy knife can be used to open the ureteric orifice and the intravesical ureter up to the 'bulge' in the bladder wall thus exposing and allowing extraction of the impacted stone. Alternatively the urethrotome knife can be used to open the lower ureter and it is claimed that this is less likely to cause a ureteric meatal stenosis.

An extended meatotomy of this type can be followed by transient ureteric reflux of urine on micturition which gives rise to some pain/discomfort in the loin on voiding. This normally resolves within a few days.

If, at the time of cystoscopy, the ureteric orifice appears normal and there is no swelling of the intravesical ureter, the floppy end of a guide wire should be passed up the ureter. With reasonable luck, the guide wire passes alongside the calculus into the upper ureter and its position can be checked radiologically. The ureteroscope can then be passed alongside the guide wire, usually between the guide wire and the posterior wall of the ureter. The modern miniscope, a fibreoptic ureteroscope with a diameter of 6.0–7.5 FG, has made the examination of the lower ureter very much easier by avoiding the need to dilate the lower ureter. The normal size of the human ureter is of the order of 8–9 FG.

Some difficulty can be encountered when passing a 9.5 FG ureteroscope because the ureteric orifice and lower ureter may well require dilatation. If the stone in the lower ureter prevents the passage of a guide wire, dilatation of the distal ureter can be undertaken using the metal olivary headed dilators or a balloon dilator. Dilatation of the lower ureter is not without its hazards. Serial Teflon dilators up to 12 FG can be used through a 23 FG cystoscope. Balloon dilators are expensive but provide a method of distending the lower ureter to 12–16 FG with a high pressure balloon.

Passage of the ureteroscope into the ureter can be facilitated by turning the instrument through 180° so that the beak is passed posteriorly behind the guide wire and under the anterior lip of the ureter. Another manoeuvre is to back load the ureteroscope onto the guide wire but this obstructs the working channel of the instrument reducing the flow of irrigating fluid and obscuring the view. Under these circumstances it is helpful to use irrigation fluid delivered under pressure. If problems are encountered with the passage of the guide wire it can be useful to load the ureteroscope with the guide wire or a ureteric catheter and then use the protruding tip of the guide wire/ureteric catheter to insert into the lower ureter.

With a stone 3 mm in diameter, it should be possible to extract the calculus using a stone basket. There are two main types of basket, namely the Dormia and the Segura types. The Dormia basket has four or six wires spirally situated, whereas the Segura has four flat wires with larger gaps to allow entry of the stone into the basket. Mucosa can be picked up by the wires when the basket is closed and care does need to be taken to avoid damage to the lower ureter. Similarly triradiate graspers which can be passed up through the ureteroscope can damage the delicate mucosal lining of the ureter. If the stone cannot be negotiated into the basket, disintegration using in situ lithotripsy with the electrohydraulic (EHL) or ultrasonic machines may need to be considered. The 3 FG EHL electrodes can be passed up the ureteroscope but considerable care needs to be taken with this machine. EHL electrodes are more readily passed endoscopically but the spark gap discharge can perforate the ureter or damage the distal end of the ureteroscope. Close contact should be maintained between the tip of the electrode and the calculus. Adequate irrigation at the tip of the ureteroscope is also an advantage and single shock discharges of the EHL are preferable.

If there was any risk that the ureter had been damaged during a stone extraction, it is a wise precaution to insert a pig-tail stent which can be removed 1–2 weeks later when the patient's condition has stabilized.

Ultrasonic lithotripsy in the ureter presents technical difficulties. The sonotrobe loses energy if it makes contact with the sheath of the ureteroscope. Pulsed dye lasers are probably the safest and the optimal method of disintegrating ureteric stones but the cost of these machines is still too expensive for most units. Other methods such as the EMS Lithoclast using ballistic energy from an air compressor is an interesting introduction providing a method of stone fragmentation without risk of tissue damage.

Treating ureteric stones has been transformed in the past decade with the introduction of dedicated modern equipment. Further developments and more sophisticated equipment must surely be anticipated making the operation of open ureterolithotomy virtually obsolete.

Case 2

A 30-year-old woman presented with the onset of painless haematuria which was total throughout the stream and persisted for a period of 12 hours. On questioning she admitted that she had noticed a dull ache in the region of the right loin intermittently over the last month but she had not taken any notice of this. In the past she had experienced two episodes of renal colic which were acute. One was on the right side which had occurred about 6 years previously and the second attack occurred on the left side about 3 years after that attack. In view of the painless haematuria she was referred for an urgent outpatient appointment. On clinical examination no significant physical signs could be detected. The urine specimen revealed evidence of proteinuria and microscopy showed both red and white cells, 5–10 per high power field. Culture showed no growth.

An intravenous urogram (IVU) was performed; the plain films showed multiple small opacities in the right and left renal areas. At the level of the transverse process of the third lumbar vertebra on the right there was an opacity about the size and shape of an almond, 6 mm in length. Urography confirmed that the larger opacity on the right was lying in the upper ureter with evidence of a moderate hydronephrosis above this. The small opacities in the right kidney were situated in the renal parenchyma close to the distended calyces. On the left side the opacities were adjacent to the lower pole calyx and the contrast gave the renal pyramid a streaked appearance.

Questions

1 How should the patient be managed at this stage?
2 What routine screening investigations should be undertaken on a patient who has experienced an episode of renal colic?
3 This patient had evidence of small stones in both kidneys. Discuss the different causes of calcification in the kidney.

Answers

1 The size of the calculus lying in the upper half of the right ureter is such that it is very unlikely to pass spontaneously. There are three potential approaches in the management of this case, namely extracorporeal shock wave lithotripsy (ESWL), percutaneous nephrolithotomy or open uretero-lithotomy, but the important initial step is relief of the obstruction to the kidney.

Extracorporeal shock wave lithotripsy to the stone in situ in the ureter is unlikely to be successful because of the stone impaction. Shock wave therapy is more effective when the stone is surrounded by a cushion of urine. Retrograde manipulation of the stone into the renal pelvis with the ureterorenoscope or by flushing it with saline via a ureteric catheter would relieve the obstruction and a pig-tail stent could be inserted to prevent the stone re-entering the ureter and to provide drainage of the obstructed kidney. ESWL could then be applied to the stone in the renal pelvis (the 'push-bang' technique).

An alternative approach would be to insert a percutaneous nephrostomy to relieve the renal obstruction and allow the oedema to resolve around the calculus. The stone could then be treated either by ESWL or by retrograde manipulation into the renal pelvis and removal by a percutaneous nephrolithotomy.

Finally operative removal of the calculus through a lumbotomy incision as described by Gil-Vernet can provide a very straightforward approach. Attempts to push the impacted stone back into the kidney can fail or cause damage to the ureter with extravasation of urine into the periureteric tissues. The use of in-situ lithotripsy in the upper ureter, particularly electrohydraulic lithotripsy (EHL) does introduce the risk of damage to the ureter. A percutaneous approach to the ureter via the kidney requires careful manipulation of the nephroscope into the upper ureter or the use of the flexible nephroscope.

The lumbotomy approach provides limited access to the renal pelvis and upper ureter. Gil-Vernet described a paravertebral incision through the lumbar fascia avoiding any muscle cutting which can substantially reduce the postoperative pain. Difficulty can be encountered identifying the ureter in an obese patient but, in a thin subject, direct access can readily be obtained. The stone can be removed through the ureter or via the renal pelvis after pushing the stone back into the kidney. The incision in the ureter or pelvis is closed with one or two catgut stitches and a drain left down to the site.

In this case, the patient was given a general anaesthetic and using the image intensifier to monitor the procedure the stone was flushed back into the renal pelvis using an angiographic type of catheter – the so-called push-bang technique. This type of catheter is passed over a guide wire, the floppy end of which can assist in dislodging the stone. Finally by reinserting the guide wire a stent can be left in the ureter to prevent a recurrence of the problem. Under the same anaesthetic the patient received 3500 shocks on the Siemens lithotripter with complete fragmentation of the calculus. The patient passed some small pieces of stone over the subsequent 3 days and a plain X-ray of the urinary tract 2 weeks later showed no evidence of any remaining stone. The stent was removed the following week and arrangements were made for the patient to be followed in the clinic for a period of 12 months after lithotripsy.

2 Any patient who presents with the problem of renal stone disease should undergo routine screening investigations for a possible underlying cause of the condition. Nephrolithiasis is normally diagnosed on the radiological investigations with a plain X-ray of the urinary tract (KUB) and intravenous urography. These films should reveal whether there was evidence of a single or multiple stones in the urinary tract. If the stone is passed spontaneously or removed it should be sent for chemical analysis hence the patient should be warned about this. The majority of stones contain calcium oxalate (65%) either in its mono- or dihydrate state with or without calcium phosphate which is normally in the form of hydroxyapatite. Stones containing a predominant amount of calcium phosphate raise the possibility of underlying hyperparathyroidism or renal tubular acidosis. Cystine stones are radiopaque, described as having a ground glass appearance but are usually less dense than calcium oxalate stones. Uric acid stones are the commonest type of radiolucent stones but rare examples are xanthene, dihydroxyadeneine and triamterene.

Screening of the patient should start with the medical and

family history of the patient. A check should be made that the patient is drinking sufficient fluids, that there is not an excessive intake of dairy products with a high calcium content or a high protein intake which would increase the purine metabolism and uric acid excretion. A history of bowel disease or bowel surgery with a chronic diarrhoeal condition, gout, renal disease or a family history of stone disease, excessive intake of vitamin C or D can all increase the risk of renal stone disease.

A multi-channel blood screen for calcium, phosphate, creatinine, uric acid, sodium, potassium, chloride and bicarbonate should routinely be performed. Hyperparathyroidism may only account for 1–2% of patients with stone disease yet it will only be recognized if routine screening is performed. The condition should be suspected if the calcium level is higher and the phosphate lower than normal on three consecutive tests. A parathormone evaluation should also be performed. A raised uric acid level suggests the possibility of a gouty diathesis and distal renal tubular acidosis is associated with a hyperchloraemic acidosis with a high chloride, a low bicarbonate level and a low, normal or high potassium. Routine urine analysis should include urinary pH, microscopy and culture. A urinary pH of less than 5.5 suggests the possibility of gout whereas a high pH of over 7.5 is usually associated with urinary tract infection. Proteus, certain staphylococci, pseudomonas and klebsiella organisms can all be associated with struvite or calcium ammonium magnesium phosphate stones ('triple' phosphate). These are urea-splitting organisms which cause ammonium salts to form. Such stones are usually associated with pyuria.

In patients who are recurrent stone formers more detailed analysis of a 24-hour collection of urine should be undertaken for calcium, uric acid, creatinine, sodium, oxalate, citrate, cystine and the total urine volume.

3 Nephrocalcinosis refers to deposits of calcification within the substance of the kidney which may be related to three main causes, namely increased intestinal absorption of calcium, increased resorption or destruction of bone and dystrophic calcification which can be deposited in dead or damaged renal parenchyma. Calcification from hyperparathyroidism, renal tubular acidosis, papillary necrosis or medullary sponge kidneys are examples of nephrocalcino-

sis. Nephrolithiasis refers to stones that are situated in the renal calyces or pelvis.

In this case the calcification in the right kidney was associated with a cluster of small stones in relationship to the upper, middle and lower pole calyces of the right kidney and the lower pole of the left kidney. Urography showed a papillary blush of the lower pole calyx on the left side, but the detail on the right was obscured by the hydronephrosis. This appearance suggests the possiblity of medullary sponge kidney which is a developmental abnormality associated with a fusiform dilatation of the collecting ducts. It is a condition which is more common in women and may be associated with evidence of hemi-hypertrophy. About 25% of patients may have evidence of asymmetry of the hands and/or feet and can experience difficulty when buying gloves or shoes. There is some-times a family history and there is an association with hypercalciuria.

Reference

GIL-VERNET, J., 1965, New surgical concepts in removing renal calculi. *Urologia Internationalis*, **20**, 255

Case 3

A 38-year-old motor mechanic was admitted to hospital as an emergency with bilateral loin pains. He had been well until 2 days before his admission when he first noticed the onset of 'flu-like symptoms with malaise, headache and anorexia. On the day of his admission he noticed that he had not passed urine.

The patient gave a family history of renal stone disease; his father had suffered from recurrent renal colic.

On clinical examination he appeared dehydrated and was in obvious discomfort but apyrexic. Abdominal palpation revealed tenderness in both loins. The bladder was not palpable and rectal examination revealed a small benign prostate. The external genitalia were normal.

A urethral catheter was passed producing only 50 ml of dark urine. Microscopy of the urine showed urate crystals. Serum electrolytes showed sodium 137 mmol/l, potassium 5.6 mmol/l, bicarbonate 22 mmol/l, urea 18 mmol/l, creatinine 800 mmol/l.

A plain X-ray of the urinary tract showed no significant abnormality. Abdominal ultrasound was performed and this revealed bilateral hydronephosis and hydroureters. The lower level of the ureteric dilatation was not clearly identified on the left side but appeared to reach the region of the ischial spine on the right. Under local anaesthetic bilateral nephrostomies were introduced under ultrasound control.

Questions

1 What is the probable diagnosis in this case and how should the patient be managed?
2 What is the incidence of uric acid stones and what conditions predispose to their formation?
3 What is the long-term management of patients who form uric acid stones?

Answers

1 There is evidence of bilateral ureteric obstruction but no opacity has been demonstrated. This raises the possibility of radiolucent stones. This, together with the family history of renal stones disease, suggests the patient may have a gouty diathesis with the formation of uric acid stones.

Bilateral nephrostograms were undertaken. A radiolucent stone was demonstrated in the lower third of the right ureter just above the right ischial spine. On the left side the stone was situated over the upper sacrum.

There is a choice of treatment in this case. The calculi could be treated by extracorporeal shock wave lithotripsy (ESWL) if they could be adequately localized radiologically, by ureteroscopy or by open surgery.

Renal function rapidly returned to normal following drainage of both the kidneys indicating that the renal impairment was an acute episode. It was decided to remove the stone from the lower right ureter via the ureteroscope as it was lying in the lower third. No difficulty was encountered passing the ureteroscope (FG 6–7.5) into the right ureter as there was no prostatic enlargement. The stone was too large to enter the Dormia or Segura basket so it was disintegrated with the electrohydraulic litho-tripter and the fragments removed with the basket. A pig-tail stent was left in situ as a precautionary measure.

On the left side there was difficulty in advancing the guide wire up the ureter and the ureteroscope would not enter beyond the ureteric orifice. Under these circum-stances it was decided to perform a left ureterolithotomy through an extended grid-iron incision in the left iliac fossa, keeping in the retroperitoneal plane. The ureter was identified at the pelvic brim behind the pelvic mesocolon and traced up to the stone. A small incision was made in the ureter above the stone which was lifted out of the lumen. A ureteric bougie was passed down to the bladder and up to the kidney without difficulty. A 2/0 Vicryl suture was used to close the ureterotomy and a sterivac drain was left adjacent to the site.

Forty-eight hours after the operation bilateral nephrosto-grams showed satisfactory drainage of contrast into the bladder on both sides. The nephrostomy tube on the right was removed under radiological control to ensure that the ureteric stent was not inadvertently pulled out with it.

2 The incidence of uric acid stones varies widely, but in Europe and the USA it is usually quoted as between 5% and 10% of all stone disease. They can arise in patients with myeloproliferative or malignant disease who are treated with cytotoxic drugs. Others at risk include those with glycogen storage diseases or chronic diarrhoeal syn-dromes. There are four types of stone which include anhydrous uric acid, uric acid dihydrate, ammonium acid urate and sodium acid urate monohydrate. Bilateral uric acid stones are most common in the Middle East when the combination of the hot climate, reduced fluid intake and high protein diet precipitates uric acid crystal formation in the urine.

3 Uric acid stones can be dissolved in dilute and alkaline urine. A high fluid intake should be encouraged at all times and alkalinization of the urine can be achieved by oral intake of citrate salts or sodium bicarbonate 0.6–1.2 g t.d.s. or q.d.s. In some patients sodium retention may arise as

a result of the high intake of sodium bicarbonate and in such cases potassium citrate can be used as an alternative. The combination of sodium bicarbonate and acetazolamide has been advocated to overcome the problem of sodium retention.

The dissolution of upper tract stones by introducing sodium bicarbonate through a nephrostomy tube has been successful but is liable to cause too much pain. Intravenous infusion of 0.16 M lactate solution can be used to hasten stone dissolution. Patients who form uric acid stones can be suspected if the urinary pH is 5.5 or less. They should be instructed to take a high fluid intake to produce a urinary output of at least 1500–2000 ml per day. By increasing the pH from 5 to 7 the solubility of uric acid is greatly enhanced. Uric acid stones can be dissolved within a period of 4–6 weeks as a result of the increase and alkalinization of the urinary output.

Allopurinol has proved to be an effective treatment for hyperuricosuria. It reduces uric acid formation by inhibition of xanthine oxidase and by reduction of total purine production.

Case 4

A young woman of 24 years who was 32 weeks pregnant presented with severe right loin pain. Initially this was intermittent but it became increasingly persistent and she was admitted to the obstetric ward. On examination the patient was in pain but was apyrexic. There was marked tenderness in the right loin.

Questions

1 What investigations should be undertaken in these circumstances during pregnancy?
2 Outline the further management of this patient.
3 Outline the changes that can be anticipated in the urinary tract during pregnancy.
4 What further investigations should be performed?
5 What are the treatment options in this case?

6   What types of lithotripters are available?
7   Are there any contraindications to extracorporeal shock wave therapy?
8   Outline informed consent for the patient prior to treatment on a lithotripter indicating the possible complications that may occur.

Answers

1   Radiological investigations should be avoided if possible during pregnancy particularly during the first trimester because of possible damage to the fetus. Intermittent loin pain in the latter part of pregnancy is not an uncommon problem and it can be severe. A limited excretion urogram consisting of a plain film and a 20-minute film after an injection of contrast is acceptable under these circumstances and will usually provide sufficient information. Pelvic hydronephrosis is not an uncommon problem in pregnancy and may require ureteric stenting. In this case the plain film demonstrated a 4 mm opacity in the line of the ureter below the transverse process of the fourth lumbar vertebra and another larger opacity in the right renal area. The 20-minute film confirmed the presence of a ureteric calculus with a marked hydronephrosis and hydroureter above this. The renal opacity was a partial staghorn calculus occupying part of the pelvis and lower pole calyces of the right kidney.

A catheter specimen of urine was sent for microscopy and culture which revealed a coliform urinary infection with pyuria.

2   In view of the severity of the pain in the loin and the hydronephrosis it was decided to introduce a pig-tail ureteric stent into the right ureter under a brief general anaesthetic. The patient was started on a course of amoxycillin at this time which was maintained at a low dose for the remainder of the pregnancy. Following this, the patient rapidly recovered requiring no more analgesia. She was delivered of a baby girl at 36 weeks and 2 weeks later a further plain film failed to show the ureteric stone which had presumably been passed spontaneously.

The partial staghorn calculus in the lower pole of the right kidney was still present but it was decided to leave the question of treatment for this until a more convenient time as it was causing no immediate problem. The ureteric stent was removed with the rigid biopsy forceps at cystoscopy under local urethral anaesthesia. These stents should not be left in patients with urolithiasis for more than 6 weeks owing to the high risk of stone deposits on the stent. The maintenance dose of amoxycillin was stopped after removal of the ureteric stent.

3   Dilatation of renal calyces, pelves and ureters begins during the first trimester and becomes most pronounced by the third. Ureteric dilatation is usually more marked on the right but this ends at the pelvic brim. This dilatation used to be termed the ovarian vein syndrome as it was considered that the engorged ovarian veins caused the obstruction but this is now thought to be due to a progesterone or prostaglandin effect. Other features that can be noted during pregnancy include an increase in renal length by 1 cm and a change in position of the bladder so that it becomes an abdominal rather than a pelvic organ.

The prevalence of bacteriuria among pregnant women ranges from 2.5 to 11% but most investigators have recorded it to be between 4 and 7% which is similar to sexually active women of child-bearing age.

4   An intravenous urogram was performed 3 months after the birth of the baby and this confirmed the presence of a partial staghorn calculus filling the lower pole calyces of the right kidney and extending into the renal pelvis. A moderate degree of ureteric dilatation remained on the right side down to the pelvic brim. This is not an uncommon finding following pregnancy which can remain a feature for months or years.

Renal function was assessed with a DMSA scan and this showed almost equal function of both kidneys with 45% on the right and 55% on the left.

5   The management of staghorn calculi presents a challenging problem owing to the range of different treatment options. These include extracorporeal shock wave lithotripsy (ESWL), percutaneous nephrolithotomy (PCNL), combined PCNL to debulk the stone followed by ESWL to break the residual fragments or open surgery. The choice depends on the stone burden, on the size of the pelvic, infundibular and caliceal components and whether the staghorn is partial or complete.

In the case of this young mother the stone burden was not large; the solitary calculus filled the lower part of the renal pelvis and two of the lower pole calyces, thus fitting the definition of a partial staghorn.

She was anxious to be treated as an outpatient if possible in view of the fact that she was breast-feeding her baby. It was therefore decided to treat her by ESWL.

6 Lithotripters should be considered in terms of:

1 the mechanism of the shock wave generation;
2 the method of localizing the stone.

There are three basic types of shock wave generators. The original lithotripter, the Dornier Human Model 3, produced the shock wave from a high voltage spark gap discharge under water. This produced a sudden expansion of water and gas initiating a shock wave that could be focused onto the stone.

In the second generation of lithotripters other methods of producing shock waves were introduced such as the electromagnetic coil and piezo-ceramic crystals. When a high voltage current is discharged through an electromagnetic coil, the magnetic field that is produced can be used to repel an adjacent metallic membrane. The sudden movement of this initiates the shock wave which passes through the shock head and is focused onto the stone by an acoustic lens.

The third type is based on the piezo-electric lithotripter which develops a shock wave from an array of piezo-ceramic crystals mounted on a spheroidal plate. When an electric current is passed across these crystals, they suddenly change shape and this movement is sufficient to initiate a shock wave.

The focal zone and the focal length of the shock wave generator are critical factors. Accurate targeting of the stone is essential particularly if the focal zone is small. The focal length is of particular relevance when treating large obese patients. In some patients usually over 16 stone (> 100 kg) the stone in the kidney may be beyond the focal length of the lithotripter.

Urinary tract stones are localized on the lithotripter either by X-rays or by ultrasound scanning. Some modern machines provide both types of imaging thus facilitating the treatment of both radiopaque and radiolucent stones.

7   The patient who has a bleeding diathesis or who is on anticoagulant therapy should not be treated by ESWL owing to the risk of a subcapsular or perirenal haematoma. Shock wave therapy is also contraindicated during pregnancy owing to the theoretical risk of fetal damage from the shock wave. Gross obesity or deformity as in myelodysplasia may preclude treatment on a lithotripter.

8   The patient should be given careful instructions about this modern form of treatment. Many are frightened by the machine and the apprehensive patient does seem to experience more pain and a higher incidence of cardiac arrhythmias.

Treatment on certain lithotripters can be painful and some patients will require more sedoanalgesia than others. If the patient cannot lie still such as in the case of a child, a general anaesthetic is required. Pain varies with the intensity of the shock wave from the machine, the number of shocks that are used and the patient. Treatment on the original Dornier HM3 required general or regional anaesthesia and the patient was immersed in a water bath. Second and third generation machines are used in the majority of cases without general anaesthesia but the number of shocks and the number of treatments necessary to fragment the stone does vary widely. Patients do need to be carefully counselled about the treatment. The younger thin patient tends to experience more pain. The patient should be warned that more than one treatment may be required. Fragmentation of the stone depends on the size and composition of the stone and it is not possible to predict the response.

The larger the stone, the more stone debris can be anticipated. As a rule of thumb, any stone of 2 cm or more in diameter is liable to produce sufficient debris to risk obstructing the ureter. Stone debris stagnates in the ureter in some cases forming what is termed a stone street or in German a 'steinstrasse'. The majority of these will pass spontaneously but there is a risk of acute obstruction and infection arising in the kidney. To avoid this complication, a pig-tail stent is inserted in the ureter to drain the kidney. The stent dilates the ureter which then passively conducts urine and stone fragments into the bladder.

Patients who form renal stones also form stones on these stents at a remarkably rapid rate in some cases. It is important that a stent is removed within 6 weeks of its insertion otherwise stone deposition on the surface of the stent can prevent its removal.

The patient should be warned that after treatment some blood and stone fragments may well be passed in the urine for a few days. The skin may be bruised at the site where the shock wave enters the body and in some cases where it leaves the body on the other side too.

Renal colic may be experienced with the passage of the stone fragments but it is surprising that this occurs only in about 10% of the cases despite the size of some pieces. The patient is normally given an oral analgesic such as diclofenac 50 mg to take when necessary but medical advice should be obtained if the pain persists. If the patient develops a temperature or rigor, medical advice should be sought without delay. An X-ray and an ultrasound scan of the urinary tract should be performed to exclude obstruction to the kidney from a calculus or a steinstrasse. Arrangements are normally made for the patient to return for a review with a plain X-ray of the urinary tract 2 weeks after treatment.

Case 5

A 52-year-old man presented to his doctor with a pain in the right loin of increasing intensity over 5 days. On questioning him, he admitted to feeling hot and cold and had experienced an uncontrollable attack of shivering immediately prior to calling the doctor. He denied any urinary symptoms but he was anorexic and felt unwell.

On clinical examination he looked ill. His temperature was 39.2°C. Abdominal palpation revealed marked tenderness in the right hypochondrium and loin with the suggestion of a mass. A provisional diagnosis of empyema of the gall bladder was made and he was referred to hospital as an emergency admission.

The striking feature of this patient in hospital was the pain, the fever and the fact that the man looked ill and toxic. Urgent investigations were arranged.

Plain supine and erect X-rays of the abdomen were performed. A triangular shaped opacity was noted in the right renal area (Figure 7). Abdominal ultrasound confirmed the presence of a stone in the right kidney and revealed that the kidney was larger than the left one measuring 14 cm in length compared to 11.5 cm respectively. The gall bladder was normal. A mid-stream urine showed a 100 pus cells per high power field on microscopy. A full blood picture revealed a haemoglobin of 10.4 g/dl and a white count of $18.2 \times 10^9/l$ with a polymorphonuclear leucocytosis. Blood urea, creatinine and electrolytes were within the normal limits. Serum amylase was normal.

Questions

1 What is the probable diagnosis and what further investigations should be performed to confirm this?
2 How should the condition be managed at this stage?
3 What are the most common organisms in cases of this type?
4 How long can the kidney be obstructed without irreversible renal damage arising?

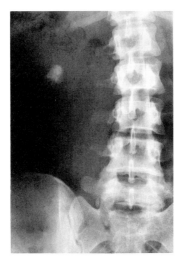

Figure 7 X-ray of the abdomen

5 How can the recovery of function be assessed?
6 What further measures should be planned in this case?
7 What complications may occur during and after percutaneous nephrolithotomy?

Answers

1 A provisional diagnosis of a right pyonephrosis was made. An emergency intravenous urogram was performed; this revealed a normal left kidney. On the right side, there was evidence of hydrocalycosis of the upper middle and lower calyces which opacified poorly. The triangular shaped calculus, 2.5 cm in length was localized to the right renal pelvis and appeared to be obstructing the pelvi-ureteric junction.

2 Immediate drainage of the kidney should be performed. This is best achieved by introducing a percutaneous nephrostomy under ultrasound control. A mid-stream specimen of urine should be sent for microscopy and culture and a blood culture taken. Parenteral broad spectrum antibiotic therapy should be administered immediately. In this case an intravenous infusion of cefuroxime 1.5 g stat was set up and continued 8 hourly. The choice of antibiotic may need to be changed when the microbiological reports are returned.

A percutaneous nephrostomy was inserted into the right kidney and thin purulent urine drained. The urinary output from the right kidney steadily improved over the subsequent 48 hours and 1100 ml of urine drained from the kidney by the third day. Culture of the urine produced a growth of *Proteus mirabilis*.

3 Gram-negative organisms are usually cultured; Proteus species, other coliforms and pseudomonas are commonly encountered in these cases.

4 A kidney can be severely obstructed for up to 2 weeks with complete recovery of function *so long as there is no infection*. Some permanent impairment of function can be anticipated when the kidney is severely obstructed for 2–4 weeks, but even after one month about 30% of the function may recover. The onset of infection with the development of a pyonephrosis presents an acute urological emergency.

5   The intravenous urogram provides a crude estimate of the renal function. The excretion of contrast indicates that some function is present in the kidney.

The ultrasound scan gives a measure of the thickness of the renal parenchyma and it also indicates if there is any evidence of a perirenal collection of fluid or pus.

Glomerular filtration rate of the kidney can be assessed from the urine obtained via the nephrostomy drainage by performing a creatinine clearance.

Good assessment of the functioning parenchymal mass of the kidney can be obtained by means of a DMSA scan. Technetium dimercaptosuccinic acid is taken up by the tubular cells of the kidney and gives a valuable estimate of the divided renal function. Following drainage the DMSA scan in this case showed the contribution of the right kidney to be 22% and the left 78%.

Under these circumstances with a kidney that has a good urinary output, it would be well-worth preserving the kidney. There is a 30% risk of stone formation in the contralateral kidney if the obstructed kidney is removed.

6   The calculus in the right renal pelvis could be treated either by extracorporeal shock wave lithotripsy (ESWL), by percutaneous nephrolithotomy (PCNL) or by open pyelolithotomy. Because the urine grew Proteus organisms which produce urease, the composition of the stone is likely to contain magnesium ammonium phosphate hexa-hydrate (struvite) and calcium phosphate which should disintegrate with ESWL. However, a percutaneous track is already available into the kidney and thus a percutaneous nephrolithotomy would be the treatment of choice in this case with a calculus measuring 22 mm in diameter.

When the urinary infection had settled a PCNL was performed. Under general anaesthesia the patient was placed on the operating table in a 30° prone position and a nephrostogram was performed to opacify the kidney. The percutaneous nephrostomy catheter had entered the lower pole calyx of the kidney. A guide wire was therefore passed through this, the catheter removed and Alken telescopic dilators were used to dilate the track. An Amplatz sheath was finally passed over these and the track was thus estab-lished. After visualizing the stone with the nephroscope an ultrasound sonotrode was used to disintegrate the stone.

7   Problems can arise during the preparation of the per-

cutaneous track. The track should pass through the renal parenchyma into a calyx which will allow good access to the stone. A nephrostomy catheter may not enter the kidney in an appropriate position for PCNL and a new track may thus be required. Structures adjacent to the kidney may be injured or perforation of the pelvic wall may occur during the track dilatation. Difficulty may be encountered with the dilatation owing to the thickness of the lumbar fascia or scar tissue around the kidney from previous surgery. A purpose-made lumbotome may be used or if this is not available a urethrotome with knife has been employed by back-loading the guide wire through the sheath.

Bleeding can be troublesome during or after the procedure and blood transfusion may be necessary. It is wise to have 2 units of blood cross-matched as a precaution.

More than one track may be required to access the stone or stones.

There are two methods of in-situ lithotripsy normally used, namely the ultrasonic and electrohydraulic. The ultrasonic probe 'drills' into the stone and sucks the majority of the fragments out of the kidney at the same time. It is important to check that the suction pump is working properly at the start of the operation. The ultrasound probe or sonotrode is a rigid straight instrument and can only be used with an off-set nephroscope. The ultrasound lithotripter relies on the vibration arising from piezo-electric excitation of a quartz crystal. The vibration is transmitted through a solid metal probe and literally drills a hole in the stone. The ultrasonic probes are straight, rigid and become hot in use. They are unwieldy to use and must be kept straight to avoid dissipating the energy onto the nephroscope thus necessitating an off-set instrument.

Electrohydraulic lithotripsy is delivered to the stone via a flexible electrode. A localized explosion at its tip cracks the stone but it can also cause severe damage to the telescope or to the pelvic wall if accidently discharged close to these structures. The electrode should be well visualized and held against or about 1 mm from the surface of the stone before discharge. The machine should be tested before use to make sure that the foot pedal initiates the required shock waves either singly or as a multiple discharge.

Failure to remove all the stone occurs in about 10% of cases but will be dependent on the experience of the operator to access the stone burden. The question is often raised whether to place a nephrostomy drain in the kidney at the end of PCNL. If there had been a substantial amount of blood loss during the procedure, it would be a wise precaution to drain the kidney. The guide wire used to develop the track can be passed through a large-bore nephrostomy tube which is then advanced into the kidney. It provides a useful method of tamponading the track. If multiple fragments were produced at the time of the operation there is always a risk that one of these could obstruct the ureter. Under these circumstances a nephrostomy tube with a long tail which can be passed down the ureter may be used.

A nephrostogram can be performed if considered to be necessary but clamping the nephrostomy, usually on the second to fourth postoperative day will soon reveal whether the patient develops pain in the kidney or not. If no problems develop the tube can be removed. Some leakage of urine may persist for a few hours but occasionally it may persist for days if obstruction is present in the ureter.

Postoperative pyrexia is not uncommon after PCNL. A routine check should always be made on the urine for infection and a blood culture. In the majority of cases no convincing cause for the fever is shown. In cases with a proven urinary infection care must be taken to ensure that the patient is placed on a suitable antibiotic cover before the operation.

Case 6

A 40-year-old school teacher was referred with a history of recurrent bouts of renal colic over a period of 20 years. She had experienced the first episode of colic on the left side at the age of 20; she remembered the severity of the pain and the relief after passing a small stone that was lost in the toilet. Three years later she was admitted to hospital for the first time with a further attack of left renal colic which was treated conservatively with analgesics. Again she passed a stone but it was not sent for analysis; examination of the urine showed crystalluria which raised the first suspicion of cystinuria. Two years following that attack she was admitted with an attack of colic on the right side. On that occasion the stone was again passed spontaneously and sent for analysis confirming the diagnosis of cystinuria.

The patient was started on treatment with penicillamine which she managed to tolerate for 8 years until the time of her first pregnancy when she experienced severe nausea. During this pregnancy she had an episode of left pyelonephritis with pain in the left loin and a high fever. After a prolonged second stage of labour a lower segment Caesarian section was performed for fetal distress.

Investigations following this pregnancy revealed a moderately large calculus in the lower third of the left ureter; this was removed by ureterolithotomy.

A further pregnancy occurred 3 years later in 1985 and ended with a second Caesarian section. Shortly after this she experienced an attack of colic on the left side and investigations showed a further stone on that side in the left ureter above the site of the previous ureterolithotomy. There was also a calculus in the pelvis of the left kidney. The ureteric stone was removed by ureterolithotomy and a percutaneous removal of the stone was performed for the renal stone. Six years later following an episode of left renal pain an intravenous urogram revealed a calculus in the left renal pelvis.

Questions

1 How should this patient be managed?
2 What prophylactic measures can be taken to prevent recurrent stone formation?
3 Are there any screening investigations for patients with cystine stones?
4 Outline the aetiology of cystinuria.

Answers

1 Cystine stones are notoriously hard. The response to extracorporeal shock wave lithotripsy (ESWL) is variable

and often unsuccessful. However in cases with small solitary stones one or two treatments should be attempted because satisfactory disintegration can occasionally be achieved. For the larger stones or after failure of ESWL, percutaneous nephrolithotomy (PCNL) or open surgery is indicated. Cystine stones do fragment with endoscopic lithotripsy using electrohydraulic lithotripsy (EHL) or ultrasound.

Initial treatment was performed with ESWL and the response was encouraging. Two weeks following the shock wave therapy the patient returned with a 3-day history of fever, rigors, left loin pain and frequency of micturition.

An ultrasound examination confirmed the presence of a left hydronephrosis and hydroureter. An intravenous urogram (IVU) showed the ureter to be dilated up to the level of the sacroiliac joint where a small collection of stones in the form of a steinstrasse was present.

The patient was admitted to hospital and i.v. antibiotics were commenced after an MSU had been taken for culture. The following day a cystoscopy was performed under general anaesthesia and a guide wire was passed up the left ureter under radiological control using the image intensifier but it would not advance past the stone fragments. Ureteroscopy was performed but the instrument could not be negotiated through a stricture which was obstructing the passage of the stone fragments. The procedure was thus abandoned and preparations were made for an open ureterolithotomy.

The patient was placed in the supine position on the operating table. An extended grid-iron incision was made in the left iliac fossa and keeping in the retroperitoneal plane the left ureter was identified and secured between slings. The ureter was surrounded by dense adhesions from the previous ureterolithotomies. The stones were easily palpated; the ureter was incised just proximal to the site of the obstruction and the stones were milked out of the ureter. A 12 FG catheter was passed proximally up to the kidney but distally it would not pass down the ureter. A tight stricture was present involving a short 5 mm segment of ureter. This was excised and an end-to-end anastomosis was performed using interrupted 3/0 chromic catgut over a pig-tail stent. A tube drain was placed at the site of the closure connected to a closed drainage system. The abdominal wound was closed with interrupted chromic catgut sutures.

The patient made an uneventful recovery. The drain was removed on the third day as there had been no urinary drainage after the first 24 hours. The patient left hospital on the fifth postoperative day and arrangements were made for the ureteric stent to be removed as a day-case 4 weeks later. An intravenous urogram was undertaken 8 weeks postoperatively and this showed good drainage of the left kidney with no evidence of ureteric obstruction.

2   The treatment should aim to reduce the concentration of urinary cystine below its solubility limit. The patient with homozygous cystinuria excretes amounts of cystine in the range of 250–1250 mg per day. The solubility of cystine can be increased by maintaining a high fluid output and by alkalinizing the urine. Patients should be encouraged to increase the urinary output to around 2000 ml per day. The pH should be raised to about 6.5–7.0 Potassium citrate 15–20 mmol twice daily is recommended but raising the pH above 7.0 may cause deposition of calcium phosphate stones. A variety of other measures have been tried. Methionine is required for cystine production and thus it was suggested that dietary restriction of methionine may help to reduce the risk of cystine stones. Methionine is present in fresh meat, poultry, fish and dairy products and few people would be prepared to remain on a diet that excluded such foods.

D-Penicillamine has been used to reduce the excretion of cystine. Like cystine, D-penicillamine has a free sulphadryl group and it can thus form penicillamine–cysteine disulphide which is more soluble than cystine. The dose of D-penicillamine varies according to the cystine excretion and it should be titrated against this. If cystine excretion is more than 1000 mg/day, 1250 mg penicillamine should be prescribed whereas if the excretion falls to 750 mg/day, a dose of 800 mg/day should be sufficient. The penicillamine is taken before meals because the absorption can be reduced by food.

Unfortunately D-penicillamine can cause many side-effects particularly affecting the gastrointestinal tract. These include nausea, vomiting, diarrhoea, anorexia, pharyngitis but dermatological problems such as pruritus, blood dyscrasias, optic neuritis and proteinuria have also been described. Fifty per cent of patients stop taking penicillamine because of the side-effects. Pyridoxine may help to reduce the incidence of these because D-penicillamine binds with pyridoxine creating a vitamin B deficiency. Alpha-mercaptopropionyl glycine (ALPHA-MPG) has been reported as an alternative preparation to D-penicillamine with a much reduced risk of producing toxicity reactions.

3 The cyanide-nitroprusside reaction for urinary cystine is able to detect the majority of cystinuric patients. Microscopic crystalluria is a useful diagnostic investigation but is dependent on the concentration of the cystine excretion. Quantification of the excretion can be performed colorimetrically and chromotography provides more specific identification of other amino acids present in the urine.

4 Cystinuria is an inherited metabolic disease associated with a high excretion of cystine, lysine, arginine and ornithine. Its prevalence has been estimated to be about 1 in 700. The inheritance of the condition involves a complex autosomal recessive mechanism in which three types have been identified. The child of a cystinuric patient is unlikely to develop the disease unless the other parent also carries the cystinuric gene or the child is an incomplete recessive heterozygote.

Reference

PAK, C. Y. C., FULLER, C., SAKHAEE, K., ZERWEKH, J. E. and ADAMS, B. V., 1986, Management of cystine nephrolithiasis with alpha MPG. *Journal of Urology*, **136**, 1003–1008

Case 7

An engineer aged 41 years went to see his doctor with a 9-month history of vague 'flu-like symptoms, malaise and loss of energy. He also had noted a backache of 3 months' duration associated with dyspnoea on exertion. An X-ray of the lumbar spine showed a staghorn type of calculus in the left renal area.

The patient was referred to a urological clinic. A plain film of the urinary tract confirmed the presence of the staghorn calculus and also showed an opacity in the region of the bladder. The intravenous urogram demonstrated the staghorn calculus to be filling the lower pole calyces of the left kidney and the renal pelvis. In the left side of the pelvic cavity the ureter was dilated at its lowest end and the opacity was lying either within this or the bladder. The right kidney and ureter appeared normal (Figure 8). Mid-stream urine (MSU) showed scanty insignificant growth; 10–15 red blood cells and 15–20 pus cells per high power field. Haemoglobin 13.8 g/ml and normal film; urea and metabolic screen negative.

Questions

1 Is there a simple method of assessing whether the stone is lying in the bladder?
2 What is the name of this condition?
3 How can bladder stones be removed?
4 Outline the management of the staghorn calculus.

Answers

1 The patient should be laid on his side and another X-ray film taken to check whether the stone moves freely within the bladder. In this case the stone did not move and it was lying within the lower end of the ureter.
2 The dilated lower end of the ureter has been described as having the appearance of a cobra-head. This is typical of a ureterocele and the calculus lies within this intravesical segment of the ureter. The ureteric meatus is usually the size of a pin-hole and the ureter above this can often be seen to distend as the ureteric peristaltic wave reaches the lower end and then to empty slowly.

   A cystoscopy was performed and this confirmed the presence of a large ureterocele on the left side. A resectoscope was passed and the ureterocele was de-roofed with the loop electrode; following this the stone was readily dislodged into the bladder. It was too large to pass through the resectoscope sheath.
3 The stone could be removed endoscopically in a variety of ways. The stone could be crushed in an optical lithotrite.

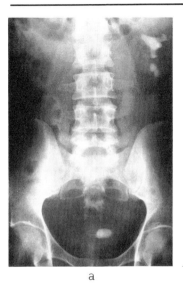 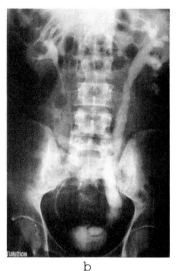

a   b

Figure 8 A plain (a) and urographic (b) film showing the staghorn calculus and the calculus within a ureterocele

This is rather a large clumsy instrument which can be difficult to pass if the urethra is tight and it can cause bleeding at the bladder neck which obscures the view in the bladder. Care must be taken to ensure that the bladder wall is not grasped in the jaws of the instrument when the stone is crushed.

The stone punch is a less traumatic instrument but it cannot grasp a very large stone. The stone in this case was fragmented with the punch and washed out of the bladder in the usual way with an Ellik evacuator.

The stone could have been fragmented by means of an electrohydraulic or ultrasound probe.

4   The management of the staghorn calculus was discussed with the patient in some detail. The function of the left kidney was assessed by means of a DMSA scan. The right kidney appeared normal; the upper and mid zones of the left kidney functioned normally. There was reduced function in the lower pole of the left kidney. The choice of treatment lay between extracorporeal shock wave litho-

tripsy (ESWL), a percutaneous debulking plus ESWL or an open pyelolithotomy and partial nephrectomy.

It was decided that a lower pole partial nephrectomy was probably the treatment of choice in this case. The patient himself however was most anxious to avoid surgery if possible so a compromise was reached. An initial percutaneous nephrolithotomy was undertaken to debulk the calculus followed by ESWL. In view of the size of the residual stone burden in the calyces a ureteric stent was left in situ and the stone was treated with a total of 12 500 shocks over three treatment sessions. The stone was cleared from the renal pelvis but fragments remained in the lower pole calyces.

Three years later the patient experienced further pain in the loin and there was X-ray evidence of recurrence of the calculus in the renal pelvis. A lower pole partial nephrectomy was thus performed.

The kidney was exposed through a supracostal twelfth rib approach. This avoids excision of the distal part of the rib which can be a cause of postoperative pain. The structures along the superior border of the rib are cleared to the costo-vertebral ligament; division of this allows the rib to be replaced downwards giving good exposure to the renal area.

Gerota's fascia is opened to expose the perirenal fat which was particularly adherent around the lower pole of the kidney. On the medial side of the kidney at the hilum, the renal vessels were identified and a bulldog clamp was applied to the renal artery.

The most important point regarding the partial nephrectomy is that an adequate removal of the lower pole is performed. It is not a major consequence whether a guillotine or a wedge excision is undertaken so long as the diseased calyces with the stone fragments are removed This can be verified by having an X-ray of the remaining part of the kidney at the time of operation on the table.

Haemostasis should be carefully checked; any spurting vessels should be underrun with vicryl or catgut sutures. Interrupted or continuous mattress sutures can be used to bring the anterior and posterior surfaces of the kidney together with interposition of some perirenal fat if this is available. The wound should be drained with a large tube drain.

Case 8

A woman of 48 years presented with a 6-month history of left loin discomfort. On routine testing of the urine the general practitioner found that she had a urinary tract infection. She was referred to the urological department for further investigation. A plain film of the urinary tract showed a complete staghorn calculus in the left kidney.

Questions

1 What is the difference between a complete and a partial staghorn calculus?
2 What is the composition of a staghorn calculus?
3 Describe the further management of this patient.

Answers

1 A staghorn calculus is a solitary stone which has a pelvic, infundibular and calyceal component. It is described as a partial staghorn when two or less calyces are involved and complete when the collecting system is filled.
2 Staghorn calculi are usually related to chronic renal infection and consist of magnesium ammonium phosphate and/or calcium carbonate and phosphate in the form of carbonate-apatite crystals. They are often referred to as triple phosphate or struvite stones. Struvite is synonymous with magnesium ammonium phosphate. Infection stones are related to urea-splitting bacteria which possess the enzyme urease that splits urea to form ammonium salts.

$$H_2N-CO-NH_2 \rightarrow 2NH_3 + CO_2$$

$$NH_3 + H_2O \rightarrow NH_4 + OH$$

Struvite stones contain bacteria and when they are broken up, the bacteria are released. The stones tend to be soft, particularly in comparison to cystine or calcium monohydrate stones which are particularly hard and difficult to fragment by extracorporeal shock wave lithotripsy (ESWL). Low density struvite stones may consist of matrix material which has a gelatinous consistency. Such stones are composed of mucoproteins, cellular debris and carbohydrates as well as the stone crystals. Ammonia probably damages the protective urothelial layer of mucopolysaccharide which consists of glycosaminoglycan. This allows the bacteria access to the urothelium which causes an acute inflammatory reaction. The inflammatory cells, the mucopolysaccharide mucoprotein and the bacteria form a matrix on which struvite and apatite crystals are deposited. Not all staghorn calculi are associated with infection. A small proportion consist of cystine, uric acid or calcium salts.

3   The management of the patient with a staghorn calculus depends on a number of factors. Careful assessment must be made of the intrarenal anatomy, the renal function, the stone burden, the stone composition, the presence of infection and obstruction. Last but by no means least the prognosis and expectancy of the patient must be given due consideration.

The principle of treatment is to achieve complete stone clearance. The available options are ESWL, percutaneous nephrolithotomy (PCNL) with or without ESWL and open surgery.

In this case open surgery was indicated because the renal pelvis was small and there were multiple calyceal branches lying behind narrow infundibular necks. Open surgery is also indicated in the group of patients with large staghorn calculi in poorly functioning kidneys which have a thin parenchyma. A percutaneous track is not well supported in these cases. If open surgery is to be performed, the type of operative procedure requires careful consideration. The options include pyelolithotomy, intrasinusal pyelolithotomy, pyelo-nephrolithotomy or anatrophic nephrolithotomy. Preoperative regional hypothermia, coagulum pyelolithotomy or operative nephroscopy may be indicated and thus should be available if required.

Surgery for renal stone disease requires good exposure of the kidney. Pyelolithotomy avoids injury to the renal parenchyma. The supracostal twelfth rib incision provides good exposure and leaves the rib intact. The kidney is approached through Gerota's fascia. The pelvis tends to be surrounded by densely adherent fat in these cases and it is advisable to identify the upper ureter first and to trace this up to the pelvis. The plane is then developed between the adventitia of the renal pelvis and the fatty tissue to avoid bleeding from the vessels that lie in the adipose tissue around the sinus of the kidney. When the posterior surface of the renal pelvis has been exposed, a transverse incision should be made to open the pelvis well away from the pelvi-ureteric junction. The pyelotomy gives good exposure to a stone in the renal pelvis or infundibula of the major calyces.

The intrasinusal pyelolithotomy provides excellent access in those cases where the pelvis is intrarenal. This approach enters the renal sinus by dissecting through the connective tissue that joins the renal capsule to pelvis of the kidney. The plane of dissection should be as close as possible to the muscular layer of the pelvicalyceal system to avoid the segmental arteries lying within the perihilar fat. Gil-Vernet described the approach and introduced retractors to assist the dissection. These retractors lift the renal parenchyma away from the pelvicalyceal structures and allow access to the infundibula of the major calyces which can then be opened longitudinally. This allows a large staghorn to be lifted out of the pelvis. Remnants may be left in the calyces which may be removed via a nephroscope or flushed out with an irrigating solution.

Anatrophic nephrolithotomy is indicated for removal of staghorn calculi from small intrarenal pelves with multiple branches extending into the calyces particularly if infundibular stenoses are present.

Division of the intrarenal segmental arteries causes parenchymal atrophy but incisions that do not transect these vessels are termed anatrophic. Anatrophic nephrolithotomy requires careful exposure of the divisions of the renal artery at the hilum of the kidney. Five minutes after administering 12.5 g mannitol intravenously (i.v.) the posterior segmental artery is occluded with a soft bulldog clamp; 20 ml of methylene blue are adminstered i.v. and the intersegmental plane is rapidly delineated by the change of colour between the blanched ischaemic posterior segment and the bluish perfused part of the kidney.

Radial incisions are made into the renal parenchyma to provide a paravascular access to the collecting system. A standard Doppler stethoscope can be valuable to identify the course of the intrarenal arteries. When an incision has been made into the calyx, a nasal speculum can be useful to compress minor transected vessels.

Under normothermic conditions the renal artery should only be occluded for 15 minutes. It has been claimed that inosine 30–60 mg injected intra-arterially into the renal artery distal to the renal clamp offers protection against normothermic ischaemia for periods up to 60 minutes duration. Hypothermia can be achieved by using cooling coils on the surface and/or ice packed around the kidney, transarterial hypothermic perfusion or by hypothermic irrigation of the collecting system; such measures should prolong the ischaemic time up to 45 minutes. The temperature of the kidney is monitored closely with a thermocouple.

Reference

GIL-VERNET, J. M., 1990, Intrasinusal surgery. In *Renal Stone Disease* J. E. A. Wickham and A. Colin Buck (eds), Edinburgh: Churchill Livingstone

Case 9

A 74-year-old woman started to become incontinent of urine. She went to see her doctor who sent a mid-stream specimen of urine to the laboratory for microscopy and culture. This showed evidence of red blood cells 5–10 per high power field (HPF), pus cells 50–70 per HPF and a significant coliform infection of 100 000 organisms per ml, sensitive to a wide range of antibiotics. Following two courses of antibiotics with trimethoprim and ampicillin respectively the infection remained. The patient was sent to a urologist for further investigation.

Questions

1 An elderly woman presents with a history of recent onset of urinary incontinence. How should she be investigated?
2 What is the difference between an acute and a chronic retention of urine?
3 What types of urinary incontinence can be recognized?
4 What further investigations would seem appropriate in this case?
5 Give other examples of foreign material that can give rise to bladder stones.

Answers

1 The history of the condition should indicate the timing and the amount of incontinence the individual is experiencing. This patient had been troubled with increasing frequency of micturition over a period of 8 months. This was associated with marked urgency of micturition, particularly when she stood up from a sitting or lying position. For the 6 months prior to her attendance at the GP's surgery she had been using one to two sanitary towels a day for her urinary incontinence. From the history the patient was experiencing urge incontinence.

Clinical examination did not reveal any gross pathology.

The general practitioner sent a specimen of urine for microscopy and culture. In fact the patient had a tight vaginal introitus with evidence of postmenopausal atrophic vaginitis. The external urethral orifice was situated on the anterior wall of the vagina in a position where it would be virtually impossible to obtain a clean catch specimen of urine without contamination from the vaginal skin. A catheter specimen of urine was obtained and this grew Proteus organisms, 10 000/ml. Catheterization also provides a measure of the volume of residual urine in the bladder. In this case the residual urine volume was only 50 ml.

A plain X-ray of the urinary tract was performed. This showed the presence of a bladder stone (Figure 9). On questioning the patient further about this, it transpired that she had been involved in a road traffic accident about 3 years prior to the onset of these symptoms. She had been admitted to hospital with injuries to her head and left leg for which she was immobilized in bed for 3 weeks and urethral catheterization had been performed. According to her hospital notes she had developed a chronic retention of urine at that time.

2   Acute retention of urine is painful whereas chronic retention is painless.

3   Urinary incontinence has been defined by the International Continence Society as a condition where the involuntary loss of urine is a social or hygienic problem and is objectively demonstrable. Loss of urine through channels other than the urethra is termed extraurethral incontinence.

Four types of incontinence were defined namely stress, urge, reflex and overflow incontinence.

This elderly patient described urge incontinence which is the involuntary loss of urine associated with a strong desire to void.

4   A cystoscopy is indicated to confirm the radiological diagnosis; the patient should be prepared for endoscopic or transvesical removal of the stone under the same anaesthetic.

Patients with incontinence should be asked to keep a

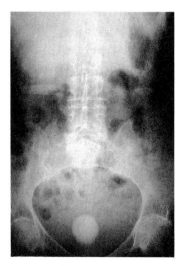

Figure 9 Plain X-ray showing bladder calculus

frequency and volume chart recording the time and the volume of urine voided over a period of 5–7 days; any episodes of incontinence should also be noted and if appropriate the number of incontinence pads required by day and/or by night. This chart is a valuable record of the individual's pattern of micturition and it is a useful yardstick by which the patient's later progress can be compared. Careful scrutiny of the chart indicates the average and the maximum functional bladder capacity and it showed in this case that she was passing only very small volumes of urine amounting to about 75–150 ml on each occasion. The chart also records how much urine is passed during the day and night.

A cystoscopy was performed under general anaesthesia. This confirmed the presence of a bladder stone about 3 cm in maximum diameter. The bladder capacity under anaesthesia was 500 ml and hence the frequency of micturition was not related to a reduced structural bladder capacity.

The stone was crushed with the optical lithotrite and the fragments removed with an Ellik evacuator. Some bladder stones can be too large to grasp in the jaws of the lithotrite and under these circumstances it is usually quicker and simpler to perform a transvesical removal of the stone.

In the centre of the bladder stone there was a small fragment of latex which had presumably arisen from a catheter that had been used during her previous admission following the accident. On looking back at the nursing notes the catheter had 'fallen out' on one occasion and she was recatheterized. Whenever a self-retaining catheter falls out of the bladder the catheter should be carefully examined to check that a fragment of the balloon has not been retained in the bladder. If there is any doubt a cystoscopy should be performed. This can be undertaken with a flexible cystoscope under local anaesthetic.

5   A piece of non-absorbable suture material can cause precipitation of crystals in the bladder. For example nylon used for herniorraphy or culposuspension may penetrate the bladder wall thus creating a nidus for stone formation.

A variety of foreign bodies may be introduced into the bladder by patients such as hair grips, electrical wires, paper clips, refills for the ball-point pens or lead pencils. All are radiopaque except candle wax.

Case 10

A retired bank manager, aged 71, noticed a deterioration of the urinary flow over a period of about 6 months. He had undergone a transurethral resection (TUR) of the prostate 4 years prior to the onset of these symptoms, following which he had an excellent urinary stream. The problem appeared to be a recurrence of his original complaint; the frequency of micturition was variable and he occasionally experienced dysuria. Two weeks before seeing his general practitioner the patient passed a blood clot at the start of the stream.

On examination the patient was a fit man for his age. There was no evidence of bladder distension but the prostate felt hard but symmetrical. A mid-stream urine showed evidence of pyuria on microscopy and on culture grew a Proteus organism, 20 000 per ml.

Questions

1 What is the differential diagnosis in this case and how would you proceed to investigate the problem?
2 How would you proceed at this point?
3 The composition of the stone?
4 Are there any other sites in the urethra where stones can be held up?

Answers

1 Increasing obstructive symptoms after an apparently successful prostatectomy raise the possibility of:

- Urethral stricture.
- Carcinoma of the prostate.
- Bladder neck stenosis or prostatic regeneration.
- Prostatic calculi.

A provisional diagnosis of a carcinoma of the prostate was made. A plain X-ray of the urinary tract however showed an opacity in the midline of the pelvis suggesting the presence of a prostatic calculus (Figure 10). A panend-oscopy was performed to confirm the diagnosis and the calculus was seen to be lying in the prostatic urethra.

2   It is usually possible to push the calculus into the bladder with the tip of the cystoscope. The calculus can then be broken up and washed out of the bladder with the Ellik evacuator.

There are two optical instruments that may be used to crush stones. The optical lithotrite has a 24 FG sheath and can be difficult to pass. Care is required to ensure that the bladder wall is not picked up in the jaws of the instrument when the stone is grabbed thus causing a perforation with extravasation of irrigant. First make sure that the bladder is reasonably full of fluid. Secondly when the stone is picked up in the jaws of the lithotrite it is important to be able to move the end of the instrument around in the bladder to ensure that it has not picked up the bladder wall. The stone punch is less likely to cause trauma to the bladder wall. Electrohydraulic lithotripsy (EHL) and the ultrasonic probe can be used to fragment stones in the bladder. The EHL electrodes come in a range of sizes, FG 3, 5 and 7. When using the EHL electrodes in the bladder on a sizeable stone it is best to use as large an electrode as possible. Care must be exercised to ensure that the tip of the electrode is kept

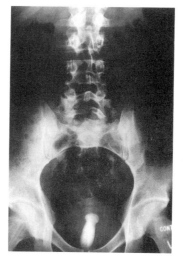

Figure 10 Plain X-ray showing prostatic calculus

away from the bladder wall and the end of the telescope as the violent discharge can cause local damage to both the tissues and the instrument. Always test the discharge outside the body before using it within a body viscus.

The EHL destruction of a large bladder stone can be a time-consuming exercise. Activation of the electrode causes a mini-explosion and the stone disintegrates into smaller particles which move around the bladder; bleeding from the mucosa can obscure the view and make it difficult to find stone fragments.

The ultrasonic probe is a safer method with a reduced risk of perforating the bladder wall or causing haemorrhage. It drills into a stone and the fragments are sucked out through the probe.

3   The stone consisted of a mixture of ammonium magnesium phosphate and calcium phosphate.

4   Stones can occasionally obstruct the urethra in the navicular fossa. They cause pain at the tip of the penis but they can usually be readily removed with a pair of forceps and liberal local anaesthetic in the urethra.

A stone can also be held up behind a urethral stricture but it is usually possible to dilate the stricture and to extract the stone endoscopically. Open surgery for urethral stones is now rare.

Since these cases were treated, new and safer methods of intracorporeal lithotripsy have been introduced in the form of lasertripsy and the lithoclast. The pulsed dye laser by means of its photo-acoustic effect provides a safer method of treating ureteric stones than the EHL; the laser however is costly. The lithoclast fragments stones by the hammer-like action of its probe which is activated by compressed air. It is relatively cheap and is an effective means of treating stones in the ureter or bladder.

The author would now recommend the use of the lithoclast for treating stones in the ureter or bladder.

Andrology and infertility

Case 1

A maturity onset diabetic of 5 years standing, aged 63 years, presented with a history of erectile failure. There were no specific complications of diabetes and he was on no medication other than ranitidine and his diabetes was well controlled. Impotence was of gradual onset commencing with less than full erections which were poorly maintained and often lost before or soon after penetration. He had not been able to have satisfactory intercourse for 3 years and had largely given up trying. Spontaneous erections were few and far between but were usually of better quality and although brief in duration were estimated by the patient to be good enough to achieve penetration.

Examination

Blood pressure normal, urinalysis – sugar + +, obese abdomen, peripheral pulses normal and no clinical evidence of autonomic neuropathy, testes of normal size and consistency and penis palpably normal with no balanitis or phimosis.

Questions

1 What investigations would you undertake?
2 What is the likely cause of the erectile failure?
3 What treatment options are available?

Answers

1 A hormone profile is not a routine investigation in all patients with erectile failure. If the libido is normal and testicular size is good there is no reason to suspect that the patient would have a low plasma testosterone level or hyperprolactinaemia. The glycosylated haemoglobin level can be checked to determine the degree of control of diabetes.

2 About 30–50% of adult male diabetics develop impotence for a variety of reasons. The problem may be vasculogenic, neurogenic, psychogenic or a combination of all of these.

3 The most useful diagnostic test is to assess the patient's response to an intracorporeal injection of a vasoactive agent such as papaverine or prostaglandin E1 (PGE1). This is performed using an insulin syringe with integral fine needle applying compression to the base of the penis and then getting the patient to stand up and apply digital pressure to the deep dorsal vein infrapubically and massaging the penis with the other hand. The degree of tumescence is then observed and recorded. The choice and dose of vasoactive agent is decided by the clinician from the history and clinical examination. In the case described the important feature is the observation by the patient that spontaneous erections were preserved and perceived by the patient to be of good quality. In this instance the response to intracorporeal papaverine (ICP) should be at least as good and care must be taken not to give too large a dose and produce a prolonged erection. PGE1 is safer than papaverine in this respect but much more expensive. If the patient responds with good tumescence or an erection then they can be taught to self inject (Figure 11) and established on a self-injection programme. The patient described responded to 30 mg of papaverine which produced an erection lasting for 30 minutes. He was readily instructed and supervised injecting himself with the same dose at the next outpatient visit and was supplied with the necessary ampoules, syringes and sterets for self injection at home. Having re-established successful intercourse he only required to self-inject on a few occasions before being able to have intercourse without the necessity of injection. It is assumed that this man's erectile failure was

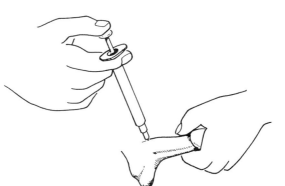

Figure 11 Self-injection

largely psychogenic in nature and 50% of such patients only require self-injection over the short term to alleviate performance anxiety. If relapse occurs then self-injection can be resumed.

Case 2

A 55-year-old man was referred with impotence of 3 years' duration. This occurred soon after medication with nifedipine and a thiazide diuretic to control his blood pressure. Spontaneous and early morning erections were observed by the patient but were of no better quality than that achieved on stimulation.

Examination

Normotensive, short stature with obese abdomen and short penis partly 'buried' in suprapubic fat. Testes of normal size and peripheral pulses normal.

Question

How would you investigate and treat this man?

Answer

It is always worth changing the hypotensive medication from a beta blocker and thiazide diuretic as both have been implicated as causal agents in erectile failure. Substitution of such therapy with an ace inhibitor such as Captopril may prove beneficial. This was not the case however in this man; although his blood pressure remained well controlled erectile function

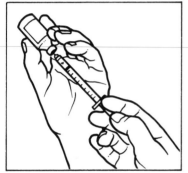

1 Draw medication up into a fixed needle syringe

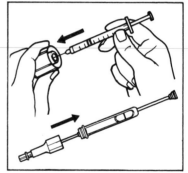

2 Load the syringe into the Auto Injector

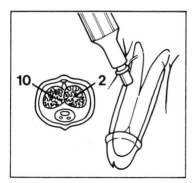

3 Select the correct injection site. Position the needle at 10 or 2 o'clock.

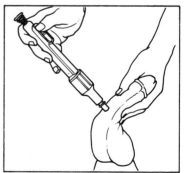

4 Locate the Auto Injector and press button to complete the injection.

Figure 12 The use of an autoinjector

did not return. He responded to 30 mg of intracorporeal papaverine which produced good tumescence in the out-patient clinic. Attempts were made to teach him to self-inject on his next visit but his obese abdomen obviated a clear view of his penis when standing. He was sufficiently well motivated to lose weight and by wearing an abdominal binder and using an autoinjector the problem was overcome. The autoinjector was specifically developed to overcome the problems of needle phobia and, as in this case, obese men with pendulous abdomens unable accurately to locate the site of injection. The autoinjector is provided with two adaptors for use with either 2 ml or 1 ml fixed needle insulin syringes. The medication is drawn up into the fixed needle syringe by the patient and is loaded into the autoinjector. At the touch of a button the needle is automatically inserted and the contents of the syringe injected. This all takes place without sight of the needle (Figure 12). The patient was then able to inject successfully and became established on a self-injection programme with a dose of 30 mg papaverine delivered by a 1 ml insulin syringe. Although he did not respond fully to this dose in the clinical setting he was able to achieve a better quality erection under domestic circumstances and continues to self-inject some 3 years later.

Case 3

A heavy smoker of many years standing aged 68 years was referred for further investigation of impotence. He had had successful coronary artery bypass surgery 4 years previously following a myocardial infarction and subsequent angina and had been impotent since that time. No nocturnal spontaneous erections were perceived by the patient during this time. In the past year he had developed claudication in the left leg on walking about 800 metres ($^1/_2$ mile). Medication with aspirin.

Examination

Penis and testes normal. No pulses palpable on left leg below the femoral. Right leg absent posterior tibial and dorsalis pedis pulses.

Discussion

In view of the likely vasculogenic nature of this man's impotence he was given a relatively large test dose of 60 mg papaverine intracorporeally which failed to produce an erection. Poor tumescence only was obtained and he was therefore given literature to read regarding external suction devices

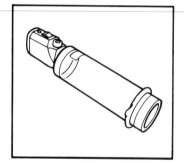

1 Slip ring over open end of cylinder

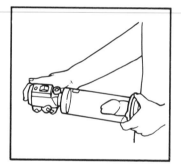

2 Place cylinder over penis

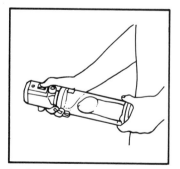

3 Switch on pump to create erection

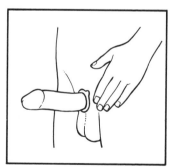

4 Slip ring off cylinder onto erect penis

Figure 13 The use of a suction device

and penile prostheses. On his next outpatient review he expressed interest in trying a suction device (Figure 13) in preference to the surgical insertion of prostheses. He was therefore shown an example of a suction device and instructed in its use aided by watching a video demonstration supplied by the manufacturers. He was given the name and address of the supplier and has subsequently purchased a device which he has used satisfactorily.

Case 4

A young insulin dependent diabetic aged 35 years presented with impotence of 5 years' duration. Onset was gradual with poor quality erections which were poorly maintained. Spontaneous erections were also infrequent and no stronger. Intercourse was increasingly difficult to achieve and was unsatisfactory for both him and his partner. Penetration had not been possible for at least 3 years when referred for investigation and treatment. He had developed gangrene of his left big toe 5 years previously which was treated by amputation.

Examination

Normotensive. Urine – sugar + +. Genitalia normal. Diminished left popliteal pulse and absent dorsalis pedis and posterior tibial pulses. Evidence of peripheral neuropathy both feet.

Discussion

The tumescent response to a test dose of 30 mg papaverine intracorporeally was only poor and this was no better when given 60 mg on his next visit. Although he had evidence of autonomic neuropathy the major contributory cause of his erectile failure was vasculogenic in view of his minimal response to papaverine. Treatment options were discussed with him and he elected to undergo the surgical insertion of penile prostheses. A range of prostheses were shown to him and his partner and after discussion the semi-rigid or malleable prostheses (Figure 14) were chosen in preference to the inflatable variety. The reasons behind this choice were from a surgical point of view a much shorter operating time and hence less risk of infection in a severe diabetic. The patient did not undertake any sporting activities requiring him to change or shower in public and hence concealment was not an important factor. The patient was admitted for surgery which was performed under general anaesthesia via a peno-scrotal incision and antibiotic cover. He was discharged home 3 days later on mild analgesia and oral antibiotics for a further week. Intercourse was resumed 6 weeks later to the complete satisfaction of the patient and his partner who both consider that the operation had saved their marriage.

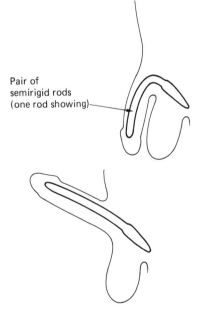

Pair of
semirigid rods
(one rod showing)

Figure 14 A malleable prosthesis

Case 5

A man of 57 years developed pain and curvature of the penis on erection and noticed that he had developed a palpable lump. Distortion of the penis made intercourse impossible.

Examination

An irregular hard plaque of tissue in the dorsum of the penis at the junction of the proximal ⅔ with the distal ⅓.

Questions

1 What is the likely diagnosis?
2 What is the natural history of the condition?
3 What is the treatment?

Answers

1 The condition was described by de la Peyronie and is named after him. It is characterized by the development of a plaque of fibrous tissue in the penis which often causes pain and almost always distortion of the erect penis usually in a dorsal or dorso-lateral direction.
2 The natural history of the condition is somewhat unpredictable in that it may improve, progress or stay very much the same. The discomfort usually settles spontaneously and the plaque may significantly alter and hence the degree of distortion on erection may change.
3 There is no convincing evidence that any of a variety of local treatments or oral medication favourably influences the natural history of this condition, although vitamin E and Potaba have their advocates. When the condition has stabilized, i.e. the pain has settled and there has been no change in the degree of distortion of the penis, then surgical straightening of the penis can be performed if the patient has strong erections but intercourse is difficult or impossible due to the curvature. If the patient has poor erections due to encroachment of the plaque to involve the

erectile tissue then the insertion of penile prostheses is the preferred surgical option. In the patient described his penile pain settled in 3 months. The degree of dorsal angulation of the penis was assessed in the outpatient clinic by the intracorporeal injection of prostaglandin E1 (less risk of prolonged erection than papaverine). The injection produced an erection and the dorsal angulation at mid-shaft level was observed as being 80° with a left lateral angulation of 30°. As penetration was impossible and the angulation had not changed over a 6-month period he underwent a modified Nesbit's operation in which segments of tunica albuginea are excised from the ventrum of the penis opposite the point of maximum curvature. This serves to straighten the penis at the expense of a little length (Figure 15). The functional result was good with no residual sequelae.

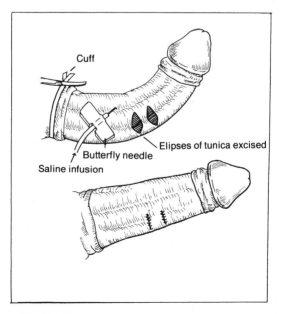

Figure 15 A modified Nesbit's operation

Case 6

A patient aged 33 years with multiple sclerosis had developed erectile failure of 1 year's duration. He was given a test dose of 15 mg of intracorporeal papaverine to test his response. A full erection was obtained and he returned to hospital 4 hours later with a persisting erection which was becoming uncomfortable.

Questions

1 Why did this patient develop this complication and how can it be avoided?
2 What is the treatment?

Answers

1 Patients with either psychogenic or particularly neuro-genic impotence are very sensitive to intracorporeal papaverine injections and unless extreme caution is used to administer a small dose then a prolonged erection may ensue. Prostaglandin E1 is a safer option than papaverine under these circumstances as the risk of a prolonged erection is minimal with this drug. Any patient who receives an intracorporeal injection of a vasoactive agent must be given instructions to return if a prolonged erection ensues.
2 If the patient returns early then it is a simple matter to decompress the penis with a 19-gauge butterfly needle inserted into one of the corpora to release the contained dark fluid blood. An occlusive cuff is then placed around the base of the penis and 1 mg of metaraminol (Aramine) or similar vasoconstrictive agent diluted in normal saline is injected via the butterfly needle and massaged around the penis. The penis is further aspirated, the cuff released, the butterfly needle removed and digital pressure applied to the site. This procedure is always successful provided the patient is treated soon enough. Delay is disastrous as the erectile tissue suffers from anoxia, decompression may not be readily achieved and subsequently corporal fibrosis develops with resultant impotence. Priapism or persistent painful erection can occur spontaneously and is particu-

larly prevalent in patients with sickle cell trait or on haemodialysis.

Case 7

A young man of 24 years suffered a severe crushing injury to the pelvis with rupture of the posterior urethra in an industrial accident. The pelvis fracture was treated with external fixation and the bladder was drained with a suprapubic catheter. The resulting urethral stricture at the site of the urethral disruption was treated initially by urethrotomy and bouguage but subsequently surgical repair via a combined abdomino-perineal route with successful end-to-end anastomosis. He was rendered impotent by the accident and was referred for further investigation and treatment.

Examination

Healed surgical scars of pelvic fixation and suprapubic catheter. Penis palpably normal.

Question

How should this man be investigated?

Answer

Impotence after fractured pelvis with ruptured urethra is usually neurogenic in nature and the patient should respond to the intracorporeal injection of a vasoactive agent. He was given a small test dose of 7.5 mg papaverine to which he did not respond. In subsequent visits he was given 15 mg, 30 mg and finally 60 mg papaverine but only modest tumescence was achieved. It was therefore highly likely that he had a vascular inflow problem and underwent colour Doppler duplex scanning of the cavernosal arteries. This demonstrated a reduced blood flow, < 25 ml/s, in both the cavernosal arteries. The patient proceeded to bilateral selective pudendal arteriography with digital subtraction. This demonstrated the pudendal arteries to be normal but there was poor filling of the cavernosal arteries bilaterally. The dorsal penile arteries filled normally. The patient is therefore suitable for penile revascularization. The most favoured procedure is utilization of the inferior epigastric artery which is mobilized, transected near the umbilicus and tunnelled through to the root of the penis where, using optical magnification, it is anastomosed end-to-side onto the deep dorsal vein of the penis. The deep dorsal vein is then ligated distally and proximally so that the arterial blood passes retrogradely via the circumflex veins into the cavernosal bodies. The results of such surgery in young men after traumatic occlusion of the penile arteries are good. If the operation is unsuccessful then the patient will be offered the insertion of inflatable penile prostheses.

Case 8

A man of 30 years was discovered to be oligospermic. He had been married for 4 years to a woman who had previously been married and had proved her fertility. They had undertaken no contraception.

Questions

1   What specific questions would you ask this man?
2   What would you look for on examination?
3   How would you further investigate him?

Answers

1   Apart from taking a general medical history, certain specific questions must be put. These should include an enquiry into whether there has been any testicular pathology, e.g.

mumps orchitis, epididymitis or torsion. These conditions can all be covered by asking, 'Have you ever had a swollen painful testicle?'. Significant trauma to the testicles is unusual but should be enquired after. A previous history of venereal disease might be relevant as gonococcal stricturing of the vasa may occur, although genitourinary tuberculosis is a more common cause of inflammatory vasal stricture in the UK. It is important to determine whether the patient has had any previous intra-scrotal surgery as the sperm conducting mechanism can be interfered with by the removal of epididymal cysts and spermatoceles and the testes may not function normally after orchiopexy. If orchiopexy is undertaken after puberty then the spermatogenic potential of the testis is lost. Always enquire whether there was any concern regarding testicular descent during childhood. The vas deferens may be accidentally divided during operations for inguinal hernia. Exposure to ionizing radiation and previous radiotherapy and/or chemotherapy would be apparent from the medical history.

2   A note should be made of the body build, whether there is a female type of body fat distribution. Is there gynaecomastia which might suggest a Klinefelter's syndrome? Does the patient shave and is the body and pubic hair of a male pattern? A detailed examination of the external genitalia should follow.

Penis

A tight *phimosis* may be discovered causing trapping of the ejaculate in the preputial space. There may be significant *hypospadias*, preventing ejaculation into the upper vagina. Usually the penis is quite normal and careful attention must be directed to the examination of the intra-scrotal contents.

Scrotum

This examination *must* be carried out with the patient *standing up* – as this is the only way in which *varicoceles* of anything less than enormous size can be detected. The patient should stand in a good light and the cord must be lightly palpated. He should then be instructed to cough or perform a Valsalva manoeuvre. This will assist detection of an impulse caused by the retrograde surge of venous blood filling the dilated veins of the pampiniform plexus. A varicocele is usually left sided but can be bilateral. Some men with a varicocele have a poor sperm count; if so then varicocelectomy usually improves both the quantity and quality of the sperm. The size of the varicocele has little bearing on the degree of improvement; hence it is *extremely important* not to overlook the presence of a small varicocele, as an opportunity to help the patient may otherwise be missed. A Doppler stethoscope is extremely useful in detecting small varicoceles. The patient should now be examined *supine* – to facilitate careful palpation of the testes, epididymes and vasa. The groins must be inspected for the presence of surgical scars denoting previous orchiopexy or herniorrhapy. The shape, size and consistency of the *testes* should be noted, together with the normality or otherwise of the *epididymes*. The fibrous thickening of previous epididymitis may be apparent in the body or tail of the epididymis. A tensely cystic and some-what enlarged caput epididymis is usually apparent in patients with obstruction at this site. An absent *vas* is readily diagnosed on clinical examination, and it may also be possible to feel an atretic segment. The irregularly thickened and beaded vas, the sign of previous tuberculosis can be a very obvious feature.

3 After the clinical examination, arrangements should be made for the patient to deliver another specimen of his seminal fluid to the laboratory and blood should be taken for the determination of testosterone LH and FSH levels.

Discussion

The patient in question was found on clinical examination to have a left-sided varicocele with an associated somewhat smaller and softer testis than the normal-sized right testis. His hormonal profile was normal. He was offered a varicocelec-tomy with an 80% chance of improving his sperm density, motility and morphology. The improvement resulted in a sperm count reaching normal values (Table 1) 4 months after surgery and a pregnancy was achieved 2 months later.

Table 1 Normal values for semen analysis

Volume	3–5 ml
Sperm density	$> 20 \times 10^6$/ml
Total sperm count	$> 60 \times 10^6$ sperms
Motility	$> 60\%$ (examined less than 2 hours after production)
Morphology	$< 20\%$ abnormal or immature forms
pH	< 8
Agglutination	Nil

Case 9

A man of 27 years was referred for further investigation of azoospermia discovered on two semen samples sent for examination during the investigation of an infertile marriage.

Questions

1 What questions would you ask regarding possible aetiology?
2 What features would you look for on clinical examination?
3 What investigations would you undertake?

Answers

1 Azoospermia or the complete absence of sperm in the ejaculate is either due to failure of production of sperm or to a blockage or obstruction to the conduction of sperm produced by the testes. In either case the problem may be congenital or acquired. In congenital obstructive azoo-spermia, Young's syndrome, because of an associated defect in the function of the respiratory ciliated epithelium the patient gives a history of chronic or recurring upper respiratory tract infections, e.g. sinusitis, bronchitis and even pneumonia. The patient will have a productive cough or will repeatedly clear his throat during the interview.

Testicular size is normal as is the hormone profile; this is also the case in congenital absence of the vasa. If the azoospermia is due to failure of production due to an absent germinal epithelium then the testes are palpably small and soft and the hormone profile will reveal a markedly elevated FSH level. The condition is commonly described as the 'Sertoli cell only syndrome'. In neither of these cases should scrotal exploration and testicular biopsy be necessary to make a diagnosis. The patient must be told that no specific treatment is available. The same holds for acquired destruction of the germinal epithelium as in bilateral mumps orchitis, exposure to ionizing radiation or cytotoxic chemotherapy. The testes are usually atrophic and the FSH level is high. Acquired obstruction to the sperm-conducting mechanism can occur in epididymitis or following intrascrotal surgery particularly excision of epididymal cysts. Accidental damage to the vas can occur at herniorrhapy or more usually herniotomy in children. Undescended or maldescended testes may have an intrinsically deficient germinal epithelium or it may be damaged by surgical attempts to bring the testes into the scrotum. Post-pubertal orchiopexy is almost exclusively a cosmetic operation as the germinal epithelium does not produce sperm if surgery is delayed beyond childhood.

2   The clinical history is therefore very important in a man with azoospermia and particular attention must be made to the examination of the intrascrotal contents. Are the testes of normal size and consistency? Are the epididymes thickened or distended? Are the vasa present and do they connect with the epididymes? Are there any groin or scrotal scars denoting previous surgery?

3   Blood must be taken for FSH, LH and testosterone levels. If the testes are of normal size and the hormone profile normal and particularly if the history suggests an acquired obstruction then scrotal exploration should be performed. At scrotal exploration the testes are delivered and biopsied. The epididymes are inspected and if they are distended with sperm (worm cast appearance) then bilateral vasography is undertaken. If it is demonstrated that spermatogenesis is taking place and there is sperm in the epididymis then vaso epididymostomies can be performed to bypass the obstruction if vasography has excluded a more proximal obstruction.

In the patient in question this proved to be the case and successful vaso epididymostomy was performed. It was assumed that the obstruction was due to previous epididymitis, although there was no clear clinical history of this having occurred.

Case 10

A man aged 42 years requested reversal of vasectomy. He had the original vasectomy performed under local anaesthesia 9 years previously during his first marriage and had fathered two children. He had since divorced and remarried a woman of 26 years who had not previously been married and they wished to explore the possibility of having children together.

Questions

1 Is it worth offering this man surgery and if so
2 What are the chances of success?

Answers

1 The commonest request for reversal of vasectomy is usually as outlined in the case history, i.e. marriage break-up and the first wife having custody of the children. A new partner usually significantly younger, who may not have proved her fertility wishes to have children and naturally would prefer them to be fathered by her husband. Motivation is usually very good particularly by the new wife.

It is almost always possible from a technical point of view to reverse a vasectomy, particularly if the operation has been undertaken under local anaesthesia. If it has been performed under general anaesthesia excessive lengths of the intrascrotal vas may have been removed and diathermy applied to the ends making subsequent reversal very difficult. If the operation has been performed low down in the convoluted part of the vas then this also increases the technical difficulty of achieving a good anastomosis. Clinical examination of the patient should confirm whether operation is likely to be straightforward or not.

2 Accepting that it is feasible to reverse what are the factors that influence the outcome? The interval between the vasectomy and its reversal is important in this respect. The longer the interval the less likely it is that pregnancy will be achieved. After a technically successful reversal it is extremely unlikely that the sperm count will ever return to its pre-vasectomy level. Between 60 and 80% of men after vasectomy develop antisperm antibodies and although the presence of such antibodies is not an absolute barrier to conception, a high titre does obviate against success in this respect. Fertility is a factor between a couple and if the new partner has not proved her fertility it is important to establish that she is ovulating by checking the serum progesterone level at an appropriate time in the menstrual cycle and that there is no past history of pelvic inflammatory disease, pelvic surgery or any gynaecological problems that might suggest blocked fallopian tubes. It is reasonable to state that there is at least an 80% chance of achieving sperm in the ejaculate after reversal of vasectomy but that the quality of the sperm cannot be predicted. In the absence of any significant problems on the female side the chances of success in terms of achieving a pregnancy are approximately 50%. Greater than this in the younger man who is reversed within 5 years of his vasectomy but less in the older man with a longer time lapse. Certainly the pregnancy rate declines if reversal is performed more than 10 years after vasectomy and is probably less than 30% of those achieving sperm in their ejaculate. It is not advisable to administer steroids to those men with antisperm antibodies due to the significant side-effects. If after reversal there is a reasonable sperm count and no pregnancy is achieved within the ensuing year then the female partner must be further investigated to include testing for tubal patency.

In the case in question successful vaso-vasostomy was undertaken with the appearance of sperm in the ejaculate when tested 1 month postoperatively. A further count at 3 months showed further improvement with a count of 25 million/ml with 60% motility in a fesh specimen. There was no agglutination and the motile sperm were reported to be actively motile and morphologically normal. The tray agglutination test (TAT) and mixed antiglobulin reaction (MAR) were both weakly positive. At 6 months' review artificial insemination with the husband's sperm (AIH) was discussed and in the event of that failing, in vitro fertilization (IVF) was considered as the next option. Fortunately a spontaneous pregnancy was achieved within the next 3 months culminating in the full term delivery of a normal child. Another pregnancy was achieved 1 year later and the patient represented himself for vasectomy.

Uro-oncology

Case 1

A 59-year-old man presented one week after passing bright red blood mixed in with his urine. He had no other urinary symptoms and no past history of urological problems.

Examination was unremarkable and rectal examination revealed a moderately enlarged benign feeling prostate. Microscopy of his urine showed more than 500 red cells per high power field.

Questions

1 What are the possible causes of haematuria in this case?
2 How should this man be investigated?
3 Assuming during investigation a well differentiated non-invasive transitional cell carcinoma is found how would you proceed with management?
4 What environmental and occupational risk factors may be relevant?

Answers

1 The finding of blood in the urine should always be taken extremely seriously. The main reason for investigating haematuria especially in patients over the age of 40 years is to exclude transitional cell carcinoma of the bladder. The commonest serious cause of macroscopic haematuria is a bladder tumour and almost all arise from the transitional layer of the bladder lining. Between 20 and 30% of patients having noticed blood in their urine will have such a tumour. If the blood is only noticed microscopically as a

chance finding, a bladder tumour will be present in a smaller percentage of patients. A variety of other conditions may cause haematuria and bleeding may occur from any site in the urinary tract from the glomerulus down to the urethra. Thus inflammatory conditions such as a glomerulonephritis, pyelonephritis and cystitis may cause haematuria but are usually associated with other symptoms. Urinary tract calculi may also cause haematuria but, again, are often associated with pain or other urinary symptoms. A history of trauma may point to contusion or laceration of the kidney. Benign conditions such as haematuria associated with excessive exercise, often called 'marathon runners' haematuria', may also be present but still require full investigation. The majority of patients with bladder cancer or less commonly with tumours of the ureter or kidney will present with painless haematuria. It must be remembered that although malignant conditions are much less common below the age of 40 years they still occur and, as a general rule of thumb, all patients with haematuria over the age of 16 must be thoroughly investigated. It must also be remembered that a proportion of patients with persistent haematuria may have bleeding of glomerular origin (glomerulonephritis).

2   A thorough history should be taken and the patient examined. In particular the abdomen should be examined in a search for masses involving the kidney, retroperitoneum or pelvis and a thorough vaginal or rectal examination performed to seek out pelvic masses. A clean specimen of urine should be taken and examined under the microscope for red and white blood cells and the same specimen sent to the laboratory for culture and sensitivity testing to exclude infection. Separate specimens of urine should be obtained for cytological examination as approximately two-thirds of patients with transitional cell carcinoma (TCC) of the bladder or upper urinary tract TCC will have abnormal malignant cells in the urine with the proportion increasing with higher grade tumours. The finding of a positive cytology with subsequent negative investigations is important and may point to an as yet undiscovered tumour or carcinoma in situ. All patients with haematuria should then undergo a radiological examination of the urinary tract, usually an intravenous urogram which will give an anatomical demonstration of the renal

parenchyma, collecting system, ureters and bladder. Some authorities would now suggest that an ultrasound of the upper urinary tract is sufficient and intravenous urography should be reserved for patients with ultrasonic abnormalities or positive cytology with negative investigations. All patients should then undergo an endoscopic evaluation of the lower urinary tract. This can be done either under a local anaesthetic with a flexible cystoscope or a small rigid cystoscope in women or under a general anaesthetic using a rigid cystoscope. The urethra and bladder should be fully examined and any abnormalities biopsied. If any abnormalities of the upper urinary tract have been demonstrated during intravenous urography a retrograde examination may be performed at the time of cystoscopy. This is one reason why it is important to perform the radiological evaluation before going on to the endoscopic study. Further investigations are arranged as appropriate and these may include ultrasound or CT scans of any suspicious masses within the urinary tract.

3 If during investigation a bladder tumour is found it will usually have the appearance of a papillary coral-like lesion lying within the bladder. These may be either isolated lesions or associated with multifocal change within the bladder. A smaller proportion of patients will have more solid invasive lesions. All the patients need a thorough transurethral resection under some form of anaesthetic. This will allow evaluation of the stage of the tumour both by examining the mobility of the tumour per rectum and by subsequent histological evaluation of the resected specimen. If the histology subsequently reveals that the tumour is of low to medium grade (G1 to G2) without evidence of invasion into the muscle layers (PTa–PT1) a policy of cystoscopic observation can be instituted. Approximately two-thirds of transitional cell carcinomas will be of this type at the time of diagnosis. Although all these tumours are malignant they may run a relatively benign course with up to 80% being kept under control by cystoscopic review and resection or cauterization of any recurrences. A reasonable approach to such tumour therefore would be to arrange cystoscopic review 3 months after the initial resection. If recurrences are found they should be biopsied and resected and further review arranged every 3 months until the bladder is free of tumour.

The period between reviews can then be lengthened assuming the bladder remains clear of tumour. The patient should be kept under review for at least 7 years from the last date of recurrence. Signs of progression including increased number of tumours, increased histological grade, or signs of invasion into the bladder wall should be dealt with more aggressively and may require intra-vesical chemotherapy or even radical surgery or radio-therapy. At the time of the initial diagnostic cystoscopy and resection multiple random biopsies of the bladder should be taken and examined for the presence of carcinoma in situ as if this is the case it will confer a poorer prognosis.

4 Transitional cell carcinoma of the bladder is one of the few tumours with well documented environmental occupational risk factors. Several factors, some highly controversial, have been described in association with increased preva-lence of this disease. Industrial exposure, urban environ-ment, cigarette smoking, dietary sweeteners (in particular saccharin), excessive exposure to motor vehicle exhaust fumes and possibly coffee drinking have all been impli-cated in the aetiology of TCC. In addition schistosomiasis is well recognized as a factor in the development of squamous cell carcinoma of the bladder.

There is much compelling data implicating occupational carcinogens in the development of TCC. Several industries including dye works, leather manufacturing, the manu-facture of rubber, paint and heavy machinery, tailoring and hair-dressing, all carry a higher risk of bladder cancer. Several specific occupational carcinogens have been iden-tified including aniline, beta-naphthylamine, benzodine and nitrodiphenyl. Workers employed in certain indus-tries and exposed to such carcinogens should be regularly screened with urine testing for the presence of blood and abnormal cells. The excessive intake of phenacetin-containing compound analgesics has also been shown to be a cause of bladder cancer. It mostly occurs in females in lower socioeconomic classes, particularly in process workers and has been especially prevalent in Scandinavia and Australia. Typically this causes analgesic nephropathy and chronic renal failure, however, there is also an in-creased prevalence of urinary tract neoplasia.

Case 2

A 39-year-old man had been diagnosed as having a moderately differentiated superficial transitional cell carcinoma of the bladder (G2pTa) 18 months ago. Recurrent tumours of similar grade and stage were present at review cystoscopies at 3, 6 and 12 months. He returned at 18 months with recurrent haematuria. At cystoscopy several multifocal recurrences were resected from the bladder and prostatic urethra. Examination under anaesthetic revealed a mobile bladder. Histology confirmed a high grade lesion with early stromal involvement (G3pT1) and carcinoma in situ at distant sites.

Questions

1 Describe the staging of transitional cell carcinoma of the bladder.
2 How should this patient be staged?
3 What features of this case would indicate a poor prognosis?
4 How would you manage this case?

Answers

1 The staging of transitional cell carcinoma can be both clinical and based on pathological evidence. The most commonly used system of staging is the TNM system (tumour node metastases). The T stage is the primary local stage of the tumour (Figure 16) and is as follows:

T0   = no obvious tumour.
TIS = carcinoma in situ.
Ta   = superficial papillary tumour with no evidence of invasion beyond the lamina propria.
T1   = superficial tumour with signs of tumour invading into the lamina propria but not as far as smooth muscle.
T2   = tumour invading the first layer of smooth muscle and bladder wall.

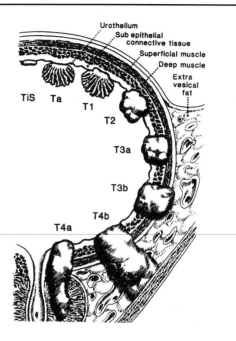

Figure 16 Staging of transitional cell carinoma of the bladder

T3a = tumour invading the second layer of muscle and bladder wall.
T3b = tumour invading through the serosa of the bladder but into adjacent organs.
T4a = tumour invading the prostate.
T4b = tumour invading adjacent organs.

The prefixed small 'p' indicates that the staging is based upon pathological data obtained at the time of surgery; without this prefix it indicates that the staging is clinical or radiological.

Nodal status:

N   = regional and juxto regional lymph node staging.
N0 = no evidence of regional lymph node.
N1 = evidence of involvement of a single homolateral regional lymph node.

N2 = evidence of involvement of contralateral or bilateral or multiple regional lymph nodes.

N3 = evidence of involvement of fixed regional lymph nodes (there was a fixed mass on the pelvic wall with a free space between this and the tumour).

NX = the minimal requirements to assess the regional nodes cannot be met.

M = distant metastases.

M0 = no evidence of distance metastases.

M1 = evidence of distance metastases.

MX = the minimum requirements to assess the presence of distant metastases cannot be met.

2 Examination under anaesthetic during cystoscopic evaluation remains a sensitive method of staging bladder cancer. This is best performed with the patient relaxed, under general anaesthetic, and should be a bi-manual examination with one finger per rectum or vagina and the other pressing supra-pubically before any resection or insertion of a catheter. It is important to note whether tumour is palpable and if so whether a simple thickening or mass, whether the mass is mobile, or there is fixity to local tissues. The next part of the staging is to take a biopsy of the tumour and then thoroughly to resect it and if it appears to be invasive to take some further biopsies at the base of the resected tumour to see whether there is still evidence of cancer cells within the bladder wall. Biopsy of the prostatic urethra should also be taken especially if subsequent radical treatment is contemplated. Once this clinical and pathological information is available radiological examination should be undertaken as follows.

A chest X-ray should be obtained to exclude obvious lung metastases. An intravenous urogram or ultrasound of the upper urinary tract should be obtained and evidence of upper tract obstruction sought as this may indicate a local invasive tumour within the ureteric orifices. An isotope bone scan should be obtained if radical treatment is contemplated (as many as 15% of patients with invasive bladder tumours will have bony metastases). Serum should be sent for assessment of liver function and alkaline phosphatase levels.

A pelvic CT or MRI scan (Figure 17) will give useful information as to the local extent of bladder tumour and the presence of obvious lymphadenopathy. Both these forms of scans will only show significantly enlarged metastatic lymph nodes and microscopic deposits will only be found at the time of surgical lymphadenectomy. Some authorities have suggested that patients who may be suitable for radical cystectomy should undergo a laparoscopic lymphadenectomy prior to surgery in order that the lymph nodes are accurately staged. This, however, is not routine practice in most units.

3   This man has shown signs of progression of his tumour in that the grade of the disease has changed to poorly differentiated cancer and there are signs of superficial invasion in the biopsies. It may well be that the grade of the tumour has been similar all along as there is some variability in the interpretation of biopsies between different histopathologists. The findings of carcinoma in situ in distant biopsies is a poor prognostic sign. The evidence from the literature is that a patient with a G3pT1 tumour in isolation stands a 40% chance of disease progression within 3–5 years if simply treated by transurethral resection. If this tumour is associated with carcinoma in situ in distant biopsies the chances of progression to invasive disease and ultimately

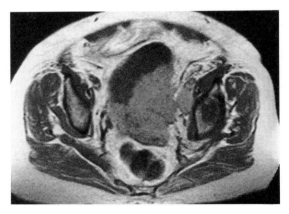

Figure 17 Magnetic Resonance Imaging Scan: transverse section of the pelvis showing extensive tumour of right bladder wall (the bladder lumen dark area) with lymph node spread on the right pelvic wall

death increase to over 80%. Therefore, this man's tumour is potentially very dangerous and may require both urgent and aggressive therapy. It must also be recognized that because of the limits of pathological interpretation of trans-urethral biopsy specimens that a degree of under-staging may take place and, in some patients with apparently superficial disease, there may well be muscle invasion that has not been detected in the biopsy material. It is important, therefore, to interpret the pathological data alongside clinical and radiological information.

4   Assuming staging investigations fail to demonstrate any evidence of spread outside the bladder a decision should be taken as to the next step in management. There is a strong argument for trying a course of intravesical BCG in patients in whom the disease is still either pTa or pT1. If, however, there is a failure to respond to this treatment after an initial course of six weekly treatments, or there is marked carcinoma in situ associated with the disease, more aggressive therapy such as radical cystoprosta-tourethrectomy may be indicated. There is some evidence that radiotherapy may be effective in high grade super-ficial tumours, however, the majority still favour radical surgery for this particular type of tumour. The standard method of surgical treatment is to perform a radical cysto-prostatourethrectomy removing the bladder, prostate and urethra, including the meatus, along with the peri-vesical tissues and local lymph nodes. The urine will then be diverted into an ileal conduit which is an isolated segment of ileum brought out as a stoma through the abdominal wall. In such a young man a cystoprostatourethrectomy will render the patient impotent due to damage to the neuro-vascular bundles which run postero-laterally to the pros-tate. There may be an argument for leaving the urethra behind if prostatic urethral biopsies are clear of tumour. However, this will mean that the patient will have to be kept under urethroscopic review for several years following surgery. He should also be offered a nerve sparing cysto-prostatectomy whereby the prostate is mobilized retro-gradely after mobilization of the bladder in order to attempt to preserve the neurovascular bundles and there-fore increase the chances of preservation of potency. Alternative methods of urinary diversion must also be discussed with patients in the younger age group. Bladder

replacement by using an isolated detubularized segment of ileum or an ileocolic segment and anastomosing it to the distal urethra is only possible if both the prostate and urethra are free of evidence of tumour or carcinoma in situ. An alternative may be to perform a continent diversion. This involves constructing a neobladder again from either an ileocolic segment or ileum alone and draining it through the abdominal wall with some form of anti-reflux device. This can be based on the Mitrofanoff principle using the appendix or some form of inverted ileal nipple such as a Kock or Mainz pouch. Alternatively, the buttressed ileo-caecal valve can be used as the continence mechanism (such as the Indiana pouch). It must be recognized when offering these operations to patients that there will be a higher morbidity and reoperation rate than with a standard ileal conduit.

Case 3

A 62-year-old woman presented with urinary frequency, dysuria and haematuria. She also had suprapubic, pelvic and left loin pain. An intravenous urogram revealed a mass within the bladder and a non-functioning left kidney. An ultrasound and CT scan confirmed a pelvic mass arising from the bladder with a hydronephrotic left kidney. Cystoscopy was performed and a solid, fixed, tumour was found involving the left side of bladder.

Questions

1 What is the differential diagnosis of this tumour?
2 How should the obstructed left kidney be managed?
3 What management options are available for this patient?

Answers

1 It is important to have an accurate histological diagnosis before embarking on further management of a bladder

tumour. The majority of bladder cancers are transitional cell carcinomas. A small proportion of bladder cancers in the UK are squamous carcinomas, a high proportion having this pattern in areas where schistosomiasis is endemic (Iraq, Egypt). Squamous carcinomas may also be evident in patients with chronic bladder irritation due to the presence of stones or foreign bodies. Squamous carcinomas of the bladder are notoriously non-radiosensitive and therefore the only treatment option in these cases is surgery if operable. It must also be remembered that tumours from outside the bladder including cervical cancers and adeno-carcinomas of the colon and rectum may invade directly into the bladder and that the treatment would obviously, therefore, have to be tailored to the primary lesion and not necessarily to the bladder tumour. Primary adeno-carcinomas of the bladder do occur although they are rare and may be associated with a patent urachus. Other lesions such as leiomyosarcomas and phaeochromocytomas do occur but again are rare. Tumours at or near the bladder neck in men may turn out to be adenocarcinomas of the prostate or ductal tumours arising from within the prostate.

2   The obstructed left kidney appears to be functioning poorly if at all on intravenous urography. It is, however, causing the patient pain and therefore it does require drainage. There are two ways of achieving drainage. One is by inserting a percutaneous nephrostomy tube directly into the kidney. This has the advantage of being performed under a local anaesthetic, however, once inserted it may not be possible to remove it and a patient with a terminal condition may be left with a rather uncomfortable nephros-tomy tube in their loin. A second method of draining the kidney is by retrograde passage of a ureteric JJ stent. This can be difficult in a patient with bladder cancer as the ureteric orifice can be difficult to find and, even if identi-fied, difficult to cannulate due to tumour invasion. A reason-able management plan at the time of biopsy and cystoscopy would be to attempt to pass a stent under X-ray control via the ureteric orifice. If this fails and the patient is symptomatic and the prognosis appears reasonable then a percutaneous nephrostomy can be inserted as a temporary measure. An antegrade stent may then be passed via the nephrostomy site into the bladder although again this may be difficult if the ureteric orifice is invaded by tumour.

Subsequent treatment may resolve the obstruction and allow removal of the nephrostomy, although this rarely happens when the tumour is locally advanced.

3 The finding of extra-vesical spread confers a poor prognosis on this patient. If the disease is T3b or less it would be reasonable to offer radical local treatment such as cystectomy or radical radiotherapy in an attempt to offer both cure and palliation to the patient. However, in this case the disease is probably T4 and management should therefore be aimed at palliation. In patients with such advanced disease radical surgery should be reserved for those patients with intractable symptoms requiring either urinary diversion or cystectomy with diversion because of bleeding, pain or urinary tract obstruction. Palliative radiotherapy may also be appropriate in these patients and a decision as to which treatment to use will partly depend upon the symptoms and partly upon the patient's age, health and own preferences. A large invasive tumour near the rectum or vagina treated with radiotherapy may develop a fistula. There does appear to be a role for parenteral cytotoxic agents in patients with advanced bladder cancer. Studies have shown that cytotoxic regimens such as MVAC (methotrexate, vinblastine, adriamycin, cisplatin) or CMV (cisplatin, methotrexate, vinblastine) can give good palliation in patients with locally advanced or metastatic bladder cancer.

When dealing with a patient with incurable, potentially unpleasant, bladder cancer, the value of palliative measures such as pain relief and psychological support should not be forgotten. The early involvement of Community Services or the Hospice movement can do a lot to alleviate the patient's symptoms.

Case 4

A fit 63-year-old man was found to have a nodule in the right lobe of the prostate during routine haemorrhoidectomy. The patient's serum prostate specific antigen (PSA) level was 9 μg/l.

Questions

1 What is the differential diagnosis of a prostatic nodule?
2 What is the significance of the PSA result?
3 How should this patient be investigated?
4 If the nodule proves to be malignant how should the tumour be staged?
5 If the tumour proves to be localized how should this patient be managed?

Answers

1 Prostatic enlargement is a common finding in men with benign prostatic hyperplasia (BPH), being present in 80–90% of men between the ages of 50 and 80 years. Prostatic nodules may be secondary to BPH or a localized adeno-carcinoma of the prostate. Other pathological conditions such as calculi or inflammation (prostatitis) can produce prostatic nodularity.

2 Studies have shown that 95% of asymptomatic men with normal prostates have PSA levels below 4 μg/l. Men with prostatic cancer would usually have higher levels with increasing levels as the stage of the disease advances. There is, however, a grey area which exists between 4 and 10 μg/l because of the effect of benign prostatic diseases such as symptomatic BPH. A large proportion of patients with symptomatic BPH and some with prostatitis do also have raised levels of PSA. Therefore, while a level of 9 μg/l may indicate malignant disease, it may also be associated with benign conditions of the prostate. The finding of a raised PSA level should simply be taken as a further reason for obtaining a biopsy of the prostate in order to gain histological information concerning the nature of the nodule.

3 The only way of knowing the nature of the nodule is by obtaining tissue for histological examination. The preferred method of obtaining such tissue is by core biopsy using a Tru-cut needle by the transrectal route. This can be done by digital localization of the nodule, however trans-rectal ultrasound probes are now available to allow more accurate localization of abnormalities within the gland and can be used to direct the biopsy needle to the site of abnor-

mality. It is also possible to obtain cytological aspiration material (Franzen aspiration biopsy) per rectum. Biopsies may also be obtained transperineally using a Tru-cut needle or transurethrally with the resectoscope if the patient has symptoms of bladder outflow obstruction.

4 A careful per-rectal assessment of the prostate would give useful information concerning the stage of the disease as a localized tumour should feel mobile, confined to one lobe and with no loss of the median sulcus. A transrectal ultrasound scan should also be performed and if the disease is truly localized to the gland the prostatic capsule should be regular without signs of distortion or tumour spread. The seminal vesicles should be regular and the fat lying between the base of the bladder, prostate and seminal vesicles should be present and uninterrupted. It is also useful to have an MRI or CT scan of the prostate in order to assess capsular integrity. The limits of all these radiological methods of assessing early spread outside the prostate must be realized and some series have suggested that ultrasound scanning will under-stage apparently localized prostate cancers in between 30 and 50% of cases. A search for distant metastases should be undertaken with a chest X-ray, although lung lesions are uncommon in prostate cancer, and an isotope bone scan as 98% of metastases from primary prostatic carcinomas occur in the bony skeleton. If radical, local treatment is to be considered lymph node staging should be performed. If MRI or CT scans show any lymphadenopathy, guided biopsies should be performed. If there is no evidence of lymphadenopathy on scanning it would be reasonable to perform a laparoscopic lymphadenectomy or open lymph node clearance either immediately prior to proceeding with further treatment or on a separate occasion. The presence of lymph node metastases confers a poor prognosis on patients with early prostate cancer.

The level of serum PSA should be taken into account when staging prostate cancer and this is perhaps one of its most useful functions. The evidence suggests that the increasing stage of prostate cancer is associated with increasing levels of serum PSA and levels over 60 μg/l are probably associated with distant metastases. Levels above 20 μg/l probably indicate at least early lymph node spread if not more distant disease. It has been suggested that only patients with levels of PSA below 20 μg/l are likely to have truly localized prostate cancer.

5 The management of an apparently localized prostate cancer must be undertaken in the knowledge that many such tumours are slow growing and patients may die of other conditions before the tumour has time to progress and metastasize. The rate of progression will depend upon the degree of differentiation of the tumour and its stage at presentation. A tumour confined to one lobe of the gland which is well differentiated may only have a 20% chance of progressing within 8 years. Conversely, a poorly differentiated tumour will probably progress in a large proportion of cases within 3–5 years and its natural history may not be modified by treatment. The evidence suggests that patients with moderately differentiated tumours, localized to the prostate with a life expectancy of 10 years, should be offered aggressive local therapy. If a tumour is well differentiated because of the low progression rate a more conservative approach may be applied, although if a patient is very fit in his 50s or early 60s local therapy may be deemed appropriate. If the tumour is poorly differentiated or there are signs of spread outside the prostate or lymph node metastases it may be more appropriate to defer treatment and use hormonal therapy if the disease subsequently progresses. In those patients in whom local treatment is deemed advisable the choice is between radical radiotherapy and radical prostatectomy. Radiotherapy, either external beam or interstitial, is used in many centres. However, a high percentage of patients will have positive biopsies at follow up indicating active tumour still present. Many centres are now offering radical prostatectomy in an attempt to remove surgically all the tumour along with the rest of the prostate gland.

In summary, a fit patient with a life expectancy of 10 years with a well to moderately differentiated carcinoma confined to the prostate should be offered radical prostatectomy. A patient with a well differentiated tumour, localized to the gland may be kept under review and simply offered treatment if signs of progression occur. A patient with signs of local or lymphatic spread or a poorly differentiated tumour or a PSA above 20 μg/l is probably not suitable for aggressive local therapy and should be kept under review and treated with hormonal therapy if a symptomatic progression occurs.

Case 5

A 72-year-old man presented with low back pain radiating down the right leg. He felt unwell and had lost weight over the previous 6 months.

On examination he was pale and thin. Neurological examination was normal apart from slight weakness in the right leg. Rectal examination revealed a craggy enlarged prostate. Serum PSA was 984 μg/l and a subsequent needle biopsy of the prostate confirmed adenocarcinoma.

Questions

1 How would you confirm the presence of skeletal metastases?
2 What potentially serious complication of vertebral metastases may occur and how should it be managed?
3 How should this patient be managed?

Answers

1 The finding of a craggy, malignant feeling prostate in a patient with back pain and a serum PSA above 100 μg/l is almost diagnostic of advanced prostate cancer with skeletal metastases. It would be reasonable at presentation to perform a plain X-ray of the lumbar spine and pelvis as this is both the site of his symptoms and the commonest site of metastatic spread from prostate cancer (Figure 18). Between 80 and 90% of patients with skeletal metastases from prostatic carcinoma have sclerotic (osteoblastic) metastases which produce a typical X-ray appearance, the remainder having lytic lesions which will produce bone destruction. However, not all sclerotic metastases show on plain X-ray and the finding of a normal radiograph does not exclude skeletal metastases. An isotope bone scan is the most sensitive method of assessing the presence of osteoblastic skeletal metastases (Figure 19), however, it must be realized that even with this method there are a small number of both false-positives and false-negatives and

some equivocal scans. If doubt still persists about an area of the spine more accurate information may be obtained by the use of CT or MRI scans (Figure 20). Occasionally, an equivocal bone lesion will require biopsy in order to establish the diagnosis.

2 The most serious direct complication of a vertebral metastasis from prostate cancer is spinal cord compression.

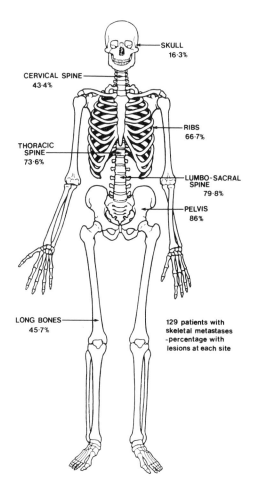

Figure 18 Distribution of skeletal metastases in men with prostatic carcinoma

Metastases growing from the vertebrae may impinge upon the spinal canal (Figure 21) and either put direct pressure on the spinal cord itself or on the spinal nerve roots. Such a patient may present with neurological deficit in the lower limbs or even paraplegia and urinary retention. If the patient has previously not had any treatment for his prostate cancer and therefore may still be hormonal responsive, active treatment should be offered. If early signs of

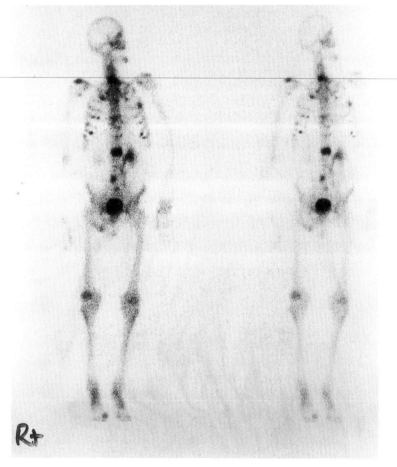

Figure 19 Isotope bone scan showing multiple skeletal metastases in the spine and ribs (black spots)

spinal cord compression are present hormonal therapy and radiotherapy to the metastases are indicated. This should be combined with steroid cover in order to reduce the oedema around the spinal cord. If paraplegia has occurred secondary to spinal cord compression surgical decompression combined with laminectomy gives the best results. This should be followed by appropriate hormonal therapy. A patient treated rapidly by this method with a tumour that proves subsequently to be hormonally sensitive may well become mobile with functionally useful lower limbs following treatment.

3　The basis of management of either locally advanced or metastatic prostate cancer is hormonal manipulation. Prostatic adenocarcinomas are under the control of male hormones (androgens) and suppression of circulating free testosterone will produce a positive symptomatic response and tumour regression in between 60 and 80% of patients. The standard methods of achieving such hormonal control have been by the use of oestrogens or by removal of the testes in order to remove the centre of testosterone production. The use of oestrogens has fallen from favour because of the perceived cardiovascular side-effects of this form of therapy. Indeed in some series the morbidity and mortality associated with the use of oestrogens has been higher than the mortality associated with the tumour itself.

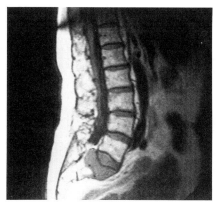

Figure 20 Magnetic Resonance Imaging Scan (sagittal) of the spine showing a metastasis in the coccyx of a man with prostatic carcinoma

Bilateral orchiectomy remains the standard method of treatment for prostate cancer and achieves castrate levels of testosterone in the serum within 12 hours of surgery. This method of treatment is unacceptable to some patients and as a result the use of newer hormonal agents has become widespread. These agents include luteinising hormone releasing hormone analogues (LH/RH) such as Goserelin (Zoladex, ICI). These cause a down regulation of the pituitary and a reduction of LH production and therefore a reduction of testosterone production. Another group of agents are anti-androgens which block the effect of testosterone at the level of the prostate cell itself (flutamide a pure anti-androgen and cyproterone acetate an anti-androgen with anti-gonadotrophin properties). There is some evidence that combining either orchiectomy or an LH/RH analogue (which effectively castrates the patient) with an anti-androgen to block the effect of all androgens at the level of the prostate (including the small levels produced by the adrenal) will improve response in some patients. This is probably of only marginal benefit and in those series that have shown an improvement in survival it has usually been in younger men with low volume metastatic disease. In patients who appear not to be responding

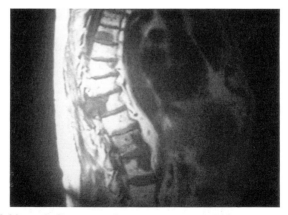

Figure 21 Magnetic Resonance Imaging Scan showing dark defects in the vertebra which are metastases from a prostatic carcinoma. One metastasis in the mid spine is invading posteriorly ultimately resulting in compression on the spinal cord

to hormonal therapy or following response begin to progress symptomatically, second line treatment is, at the moment, of little benefit. Symptomatic relief can be offered with analgesics or palliative radiotherapy to painful metastases.

Case 6

A 28-year-old man had noticed a painless swelling of the right testicle 6 weeks before referral. This had failed to resolve despite a course of antibiotics.

Questions

1 What is the differential diagnosis?
2 How should this patient be investigated?
3 Discuss the differences between the two common types of testicular malignancy.
4 How should testicular cancer be managed?

Answers

1 At the top of any list of differential diagnoses of a swelling within the scrotum in a man in the second to fifth decade of life must be a testicular tumour. The swelling, if arising from the testicle, must be treated as a probable cancer of the testicle. Also on the list of differential diagnoses should be benign cystic lesions such as a hydrocele or an epididymal cyst, and inguinal herniae should also be excluded.
2 The patient should be examined both standing and lying down and the scrotum transilluminated. If the swelling appears to be arising from the testicle, indeed if there is any doubt at all of a swelling within the scrotum, an ultrasound scan should be performed. A testicular tumour will appear as a solid mass arising within or from the testicle. Blood should be drawn for full blood count, liver function tests and serum markers for testicular teratoma (beta

human chorionic gonadotrophin and alpha fetoprotein). A chest X-ray should be performed.

If an ultrasound scan suggests a testicular tumour or doubt persists following initial investigations, the next step in the management is to explore the testicle through a groin incision. In this way the spermatic cord can be identified and occluded with a soft clamp before any further procedure is undertaken. The testicle can then be delivered into the inguinal wound and examined. The occlusion of the spermatic cord will prevent dissemination of tumour cells upon handling the testicle. If a tumour appears present the testicle should be removed through the groin incision. Under no circumstances should the testicle be removed through the scrotum as this will risk disseminating the tumour in a different area of lymphatic spread to that which the testicle normally drains. If doubt exists at the time of exploration as to the nature of the testicular lesion a frozen section biopsy can be taken while the cord remains clamped. In general, however, if there is doubt it is usually better to remove the testicle.

3   Two common types of testicular cancer are teratoma and seminoma. In addition a small proportion of such tumours show a mixed teratomatous and seminomatous pattern. The main difference of note between these two types of tumours is that teratomas secrete tumour markers such as alpha fetoprotein (AFP) and beta humanchorionic gonadotrophin (HCG); these markers aid the staging and management of teratomas. It must be remembered that 10–15% of teratomas do not produce the serum markers. It may be because their serum levels are below the level of detection in very low volume disease and has led some authors to suggest that blood should be taken directly from the spermatic cord during orchiectomy to assess the presence of markers in the local environment of the tumour which may not be detected in the general circulation.

Lymphomas of the testes do occur in older men. Secondary tumours of the testicle may also occur although they are rare.

4   The management of testicular cancer depends in part upon the type of tumour and in part upon its stage. The propensity to metastasize seems to be lower for seminomas and when they do progress they seem to follow a step-wise pattern of spread. The usual method of managing clinically

stage 1 seminoma has been to remove the testicle and then irradiate the infradiaphragmatic, para-aortic and ipsilateral pelvic lymph nodes. Relapse rates are usually less than 2% and the majority of such patients can be cured with chemotherapy. Several surveillance studies for seminoma have demonstrated relapse rates in the 15–20% range which suggests that a large number of such patients are being irradiated unnecessarily. Recent studies have suggested that patients with clinically stage 1 seminoma can be kept under review following orchidectomy and salvaged with radiation therapy and/or chemotherapy. Patients with more advanced seminoma, particularly stage 3 and stage 4 disease, should be given a course of chemotherapy as seminoma is highly sensitive to drug combinations containing cisplatin. If a residual para-aortic mass remains after a course of chemotherapy some authors would suggest surgical excision, while others recommend adjuvant radiotherapy. In many cases this residual mass will contain inactive tissue.

If a teratoma is clinically stage 1, approximately 70% of such patients would be cured by orchiectomy. A variety of methods have been used to effect cure in the remaining 30% of patients. Orchiectomy is probably not curative in this group of patients because microscopic spread has occurred to the retroperitoneal lymph nodes. The standard approach to the initial management of such patients in the USA has been to perform a retroperitoneal lymph node dissection thus removing all the lymph node containing tissue around the major vessels in the retroperitoneum.

An alternative approach to such patients is lymph node irradiation which is more standard practice within the UK. To offer either method of management to all patients with clinical stage 1 teratoma means that the 70% of patients cured by orchiectomy alone are also going to have unnecessary treatment. Some groups have suggested that stage 1 teratoma can be treated simply by orchiectomy and then kept under close review. Patients showing evidence of disease recurrence either because of an increase in tumour markers or CT evidence of lymphadenopathy can be salvaged using radiotherapy. If a teratoma has advanced beyond clinical stage 1 at diagnosis, chemotherapy will be used and approximately 20–25% of patients will still have residual undifferentiated tumour present in the retroperitoneum after chemotherapy or chemotherapy combined with radiotherapy. If a residual mass remains following treatment surgical excision should be undertaken. In 70% of cases the residual masses will be in para-aortic lymph nodes, in 18% in the chest and in 12% both above and below the diaphragm. The results of such surgery would in part depend upon the presence of active tumour within the excised residual mass. In patients with active tumour 50% will be salvaged by excision of their residual mass.

Case 7

A 59-year-old man presented with haematuria, weight loss and right loin pain. Abdominal examination revealed a mass in the right loin which moved with respiration. An intravenous urogram showed a large mass arising from the upper pole of the right kidney.

Questions

1 What is the differential diagnosis of the mass?
2 How should investigation proceed?
3 How should the patient be managed?

Answers

1 The differential diagnosis of a mass arising from the right kidney should include both benign and malignant lesions. Benign renal cysts are common and should easily be delineated by ultrasound scans. If there is any doubt as to the nature of the cysts or it contains solid elements, the cyst can be punctured under ultrasound control and fluid aspirated for cytological examination. If the cyst fails to resolve following aspiration or cytological abnormalities are found it may be considered to be malignant. Hydro-nephrotic kidneys secondary to long-standing congenital

pelvi-ureteric junction obstruction may present as a renal mass. The dilatation in this case will be of the collecting system with very little residual parenchyma. Benign tumours of the kidney are rare and all solid lesions are malignant until proved otherwise. Malignant lesions may be primary or secondary with the kidney being a common site for metastatic spread. Primary malignancies of the kidney are usually renal cell carcinomas, however, transitional cell carcinomas and adult Wilms' tumours may be found. In addition angio-myolipomas may be found and will have distinctive clinical and radiological features. Both renal cell carcinomas and angio-myolipomas may be found in association with congenital conditions such as von Hippel-Lindau syndrome.

2 The intravenous urogram is an essential initial investigation both to delineate the lesion itself and to assess contralateral renal function. An ultrasound scan will allow the differentiation to be made between a solid (and therefore probably malignant lesion) and a cystic (and therefore probably benign) lesion. The inferior vena cava should also be ultrasounded as renal tumours may either press upon the inferior vena cava or tumour itself may grow along the renal vein into the lumen of the inferior vena cava. If there is any suggestion of vena caval involvement echo cardiography should be used to assess potential propagation of the thrombus into the supra-diaphragmatic cava or atrium. In addition an MRI scan in coronal section may be of value in assessing the level of thrombus within the vena cava. All patients should have either a CT scan or an MRI scan of the kidney to assess local stage including potential renal vein or vena caval involvement, lymph node enlargement or spread into adjacent perirenal fat or other organs. If doubt persists as to the nature of a solid lesion percutaneous biopsy under ultrasound or CT guidance may be indicated. This procedure is not routinely used. Arteriography was a routine procedure in all patients with renal cell carcinoma about to undergo surgery, however, it is now reserved for equivocal cases or cases in whom renal preserving surgery is to be performed. A search for distant metastases should include a chest X-ray and liver function tests. The use of isotope bone scans or liver ultrasound is not of routine value as the pick-up rate will be low.

3   The standard management of apparently localized renal cell carcinoma is by radical nephrectomy. This can be performed either via an anterior transperitoneal approach, via a loin incision or by a transthoracic approach. The anterior approach has the advantage of being able to control the renal vein and artery before mobilizing the tumour itself with the attendant risk of shedding tumour cells into the circulation. The transthoracic approach is useful for large upper pole tumours as it allows extra exposure to the renal vessels. It may also be of value if the inferior vena cava requires exploration for removal of tumour thrombus.

There is some evidence that extensive retro-peritoneal lymphadenectomy may improve survival in cases with no obvious lymphadenopathy. In others words if there is no clinical evidence of lymph node metastases a group of patients with micro-metastases may benefit from this extensive procedure. This is still under evaluation and is not routine practice. Localized tumours within the kidney may be treated by simple excision of the tumour (tumourectomy) or partial nephrectomy. Several recent series have suggested that survival rates are as good as radical nephrectomy and this procedure should be considered in patients with early intracapsular tumours.

The value of nephrectomy in more advanced disease especially in patients with metastases is debatable. It used to be common practice to remove primary renal cell carcinomas with distant metastases in the hope that they would regress. The incidence of metastatic or tumour regression following nephrectomy is extremely low and many such reports are at best anecdotal. It may well be valid to remove the primary renal tumour if a single peripheral lung metastasis or bone metastasis is present and combine the procedure with excision of the metastasis as long-term survival has been reported in many cases with a single metastasis. It is also acceptable to perform nephrectomy for symptomatic reasons in patients with metastases if they are getting pain or bleeding from a kidney. Alternatives to nephrectomy should be considered including embolization of the kidney. If the metastatic bulk is small (if the metastatic volume is less than the volume of the primary tumour) it may also be valid to remove the kidney and to treat the metastatic disease with immunotherapy such as interferon. These modalities are still the subject of clinical trials.

Case 8

A 58-year-old woman presented with left loin pain and haematuria. Intravenous urogram showed a filling defect in the left ureter. Urine was sent for cytological examination and this contained cells from a well to moderately differentiated transitional cell carcinoma.

Questions

1 How would you further investigate this woman?
2 How would you manage the patient?

Answers

1 Findings of a filling defect in the ureter with positive urine cytology are highly suggestive of a transitional cell carcinoma within the left ureter or renal pelvis. A cystoscopy is essential to assess the lower urinary tract as transitional tumours may also occur within the bladder. If the bladder is free of tumours during the same procedure a left retrograde ureterogram should be performed. This will confirm the diagnosis of tumour within the ureter and also give some idea of both the level and extent of the tumour. It may also be useful to perform a ureteroscopy during the same examination to visualize directly the tumour and to take biopsies to allow assessment of its differentiation. Further radiological investigations such as CT or MRI scanning are not usually helpful in this situation.
2 The standard method of managing a transitional cell carcinoma of the upper urinary tract is by performing a nephro-ureterectomy. Initially a loin incision is made and the kidney mobilized, the wound is then closed and the patient turned into a supine position. A Pfannenstiel incision is

made to expose the bladder which is opened, the appropriate ureteric orifice circumcised and then closed. The kidney and ureter are then delivered through the second incision. Several authors have suggested that the lower end of the ureter can be dealt with endoscopically thus removing the need for a second incision. This can be achieved by resecting the ureteric orifice endoscopically. However, some authors have expressed concern over this procedure and suggested that it may result in incomplete excision of potentially malignant ureteric tissue and a higher rate of local recurrence within the bladder wall.

There has been a lot of interest recently in conservative approaches to upper tract transition cell tumours. If the tumour is of well to moderate differentiation and apparently localized, local excision can be achieved with little risk of local recurrence. A tumour in the lower third of the ureter can be treated by lower ureterectomy and re-implantation of the ureter either directly into the bladder or into a Boari flap. A mid-third ureteric tumour can be excised with end-to-end anastomosis of the ureter over a JJ stent. There have been some reports of tumours in the ureter being treated endoscopically via a ureteroscope either by diathermy coagulation or by the use of a laser. In addition some groups have gained percutaneous access to the kidney or upper ureter and resected tumours in this area without resorting to nephrectomy.

Case 9

A 52-year-old man presented with an ulcerating lesion on the glans penis. He had not been circumcized. There were palpable lymph nodes in his right groin.

Questions

1 What is a differential diagnosis of this lesion?
2 Where would you expect metastases from a carcinoma of the penis to occur?
3 How would you manage this lesion?

Answers

1 Benign lesions of the penis including cysts, angiomas, fibromas, neuromas and lipomas may occur. Cutaneous naevi may also occur on the skin of the penis. These lesions will not be ulcerated. Balanitis xerotica obliterans occurs as a white patch on the prepuce or glans that extends to and around the urethral meatus and occasionally into the navicular fossa. This may ultimately result in thickening and phimosis as the prepuce scars.

   A variety of uncommon pre-malignant and malignant conditions can occur on the penis. Leukoplakia will appear as a sharply defined white cutaneous plaque. Condyloma acuminatum are typically soft friable papillary lesions which may also be termed venereal or genital warts. Some authors believe that they may be pre-malignant. Kaposi's sarcoma may also occur on the penis. Ultimately an ulcerated lesion in an older man on the glans penis is likely to be a squamous cell carcinoma and this is the condition which must be excluded. Malignant melonomas of the penis may also occur.

2 Carcinoma of the penis usually begins with a small lesion which gradually extends to involve the entire glans, shaft and corpora. The lesion may initially be papillary and exophytic or flat and ulcerative. If it remains untreated penile autoamputation may eventually occur. Buck's fascia acts as a temporary natural barrier protecting the corporal body from invasion by the neoplasm. When Buck's fascia and the tunica albuginea is penetrated, invasion of the vascular corpora may occur and this will establish the potential for vascular dissemination. Urethra and bladder involvement is rare.

   Metastases to the regional femoral and illiac nodes represent the earliest route of dissemination from penile carcinoma. Metastatic enlargement of the regional nodes will eventually lead to skin necrosis, cross infection and ultimately death from sepsis or haemorrhage secondary to erosion into the femoral vessels. Distant metastases, presenting clinically, from squamous carcinoma of the penis are rare occurring in only 1–10% of such patients. If they do occur, they are likely to be in the lung, liver or bone and appear late in the course of the disease.

3 The diagnosis must be made by biopsying the ulcerated

lesion. This should confirm the presence of squamous cell carcinoma with keratinization, epithelial cell formation and varying degrees of mitotic activity. Invasive lesions will penetrate the basement membrane and surrounding structures. Most malignancies of the penis will be low grade. All patients should undergo a full physical examination and if palpable lymph nodes are present in the groin, they should be biopsied or fine needle aspirations performed for cytological examination.

The treatment of the primary squamous cell carcinoma of the penis is amputation either partial or total of the penis. In certain selected cases with small lesions involving only the prepuce, complete tumour excision may be accomplished by circumcision. Circumcision alone, however, is frequently followed by tumour recurrence. For lesions involving the glans and the distal shaft, even when apparently superficial, partial amputation with a 2 cm margin proximal to the tumour should be performed. If the proximal penile shaft is involved by malignancy, total amputation of the penis is performed.

Radiation therapy is used in certain centres in an attempt to preserve penile structure and function. Squamous cell carcinoma, however, is characteristically radio-resistant and the dose necessary to sterilize deeply infiltrating penile tumours may also result in damage to the urethra and radiation necrosis.

If there is evidence of tumour spread to local inguinal nodes, consideration should be given to block dissection following treatment to the primary lesion. Radiotherapy has been used as an alternative treatment in this group of patients.

Incontinence and voiding dysfunction

Case 1

A 3-month-old male child, who had been born with a lumbo-sacral myelomeningocele closed in the neonatal period by the neurosurgeons, had been referred by the paediatricians for a urological opinion.

On examination the child appeared healthy and lively. Examination of the external genitalia revealed retracted testes and the foreskin had somewhat limited mobility. Abdominal examination was normal. During physical examination the child could be seen to move his legs.

Questions

1 What would be the other crucial parts of the physical examination that may guide in future urological assessment and management?
2 What investigations are required at this initial presentation?
3 How should the child be followed up?
4 What urological problems may be encountered by this child over the next few years?

Answers

1 Examination of the perineal area is essential. The nerve supply to the perineum is sacral segments 2, 3 and 4 with S4 being centred on the anus. In a small child it is possible to assess sensation by observing the child's behaviour during attempted rectal examination. The anal reflex can be assessed by stroking the perianal region with the finger

tip or perhaps by scratching or pricking with a needle. In assessing the anal reflex there should be an almost immediate contraction of the anal sphincter and the description of the anus 'winking' is quite apt. On rectal examination the anal reflex may again be demonstrated and even felt, but the main object is to assess anal tone. Normally after removing the examining finger from the rectum the anus will immediately contract and close.

This child seemed unaware of the examining finger, there was no demonstrable anal reflex and anal tone was reduced. When the finger was removed from the rectum the anal canal gaped revealing the dark red colour of the rectal mucosa in the upper part of the canal. Hence this examination was abnormal in all respects suggesting that either the disease process or the surgical procedure had left a neurological defect. As the nerve supply of the bladder, urethra and rectum canal are also the sacral segments S2–4, then it can be anticipated that this child will not void urine or faeces normally.

2 Base line imaging of the urinary tract is essential. An intravenous pyelogram (IVP) provides anatomical information and some idea about function. The relevant features to note are: on the plain film, it will often be noted that the child is constipated, a bladder shadow may be visible in the pelvis, and the bony defect characteristic of myelomeningocele will be seen. On the nephrogram film the outline of the kidneys should be seen and compared one with the other. Reflux nephropathy may show itself as an indentation in the outer margin of the nephrogram, usually in the upper or lower poles of the kidney (the most common site of compound papillae). On the 5 to 30 minute films the calyces should be outlined and their shape noted. Reflux nephropathy will show itself as clubbed calyces close to the peripheral defect noted on the nephrogram, delayed function is of obvious significance as is no function. The presence of dye in the ureters and ureteric size are important as is dilatation of the ureters, renal pelvis and calyces and will suggest obstruction to the upper tracts. On the later film of the IVP the bladder should be visualized; unless the bladder is large, bladder size is difficult to interpret when the patient cannot void on command. In the case of this child the intravenous pyelogram was entirely normal.

An argument can be put for doing ultrasound rather than intravenous pyelography as information can be gained about the kidney parenchyma together with some evidence of dilatation of the calyces and pelvis but no significant anatomical information about the ureters. Hence it seems justified to perform an early IVP in these children who will remain under long-term surveillance.

Other investigations which should be done are basic tests, such as haemoglobin and serum creatinine.

3 Close urological follow up into adult life is mandatory. Follow up should consist of 6-monthly ultrasound examinations of the upper tracts and bladder together with regular physical examination to determine whether a palpable bladder develops. Formerly regular IVPs were performed, but with the advent of high quality ultrasound this can no longer be justified. However, an IVP is justified if, for any reason, it is not possible to visualize the kidneys ultrasonically. If the child fails to achieve continence at a stage when most children would be dry, that is around the age of 6 years, then video urodynamics are indicated. The video urodynamics provide simultaneous anatomical and functional information concerning the behaviour of the urethra and bladder during both the filling and voiding phases of micturition, for example, vesico-urethral reflux.

4 As implied in the previous paragraph the management of the bladder in the years 1–6 is expectant. Some spina bifida children will begin to achieve daytime and then nighttime continence. However, most will not, due to the vesico-urethral dysfunction. If the upper tracts have remained satisfactory and the bladder has not become palpable, active intervention should be considered around the age of 6.

The main bladder abnormality is detrusor overactivity during the filling phase of micturition. Overactivity can be in the form of detrusor contractions occurring through filling, that is, detrusor instability (Figure 22), also known as detrusor hyperreflexia in patients such as this child with a neurological cause for detrusor overactivity. The second way in which detrusor overactivity shows itself is reduced bladder compliance. Compliance describes the relationship between bladder pressure and bladder volume. In normal bladder function the bladder pressure changes very little from empty to full; in reduced compliance there is a slow increase in pressure throughout bladder filling.

In myelomeningocele the classic urethral abnormality is known as static distal sphincter obstruction. In this condition the patient has the worse of both worlds in that urethral function is inadequate during filling resulting in genuine stress incontinence and fails to relax during voiding preventing proper bladder emptying. Hence the word 'static' refers to a sphincter which 'sits there and does nothing'! This condition is somewhat different from detrusor-sphincter–dyssynergia which is found most classically in the patient who has suffered the spinal cord injury (see Case 5).

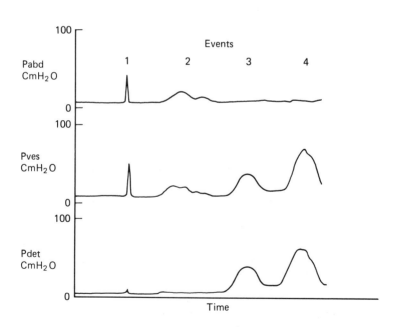

Figure 22 Filling cystometrogram recording rectal pressure (P_{abd}), intravesical pressure (P_{ves}) and detrusor pressure (electronically derived, $P_{det} = P_{ves} - P_{abd}$). Event 1 is a cough, event 2 is abdominal straining and events 3 and 4 are uninhibited bladder contractions known as detrusor instability

Intervention at the age of 6 years most frequently consists of a trial of intermittent catheterization (IC) which is usually practised initially by the parent or guardian and, as soon as possible, performed by the patient himself. IC for success, depends on an adequate bladder capacity and adequate urethral function to hold urine during the filling phase. At this age IC is usually successful and often because there is reduced urethral sensation. The main failure of IC is leaking between catheterizations. Most families consider a dry interval of 2–3 hours very satisfactory but clearly, if it is much less than this, IC loses its point. The main reasons for failure are detrusor overactivity and or urethral sphincter weakness.

At this stage, if urodynamics have not been previously performed, they should be carried out in order to identify the cause of IC failure. If failure is due to detrusor overactivity then anticholinergic therapy, such as oxybutynin (dose 2.5 mg two to three times daily), or propanthiline (15 mg three to four times daily plus or minus imipramine 12.5 mg twice daily) should be tried. If urethral sphincter weakness is a significant component to IC failure the effect of phenylpropanolamine (50 mg twice daily) can be tried although its effect is usually marginal.

If IC is not practicable then female patients have to stay in pads and pants while male children are likely to use, initially a flange external urinary collection device, before going onto a condom collection device once adequate penile size has developed.

Many patients can continue to be managed by IC with or without anticholinergics for the rest of their lives. However, all patients require regular upper tract monitoring and control of urinary infections which, if bladder emptying is complete, are not usually a problem. If the child remains incontinent despite IC and drug therapy, then definitive surgery is normally postponed until puberty. At that stage urodynamics should be repeated to reassess the situation. The detrusor and urethra must be considered separately. Uncontrolled detrusor overactivity makes bladder augmentation by ileocystoplasty frequently necessary. If there is also urethral sphincter weakness then in girls, colposuspension or insertion of an artificial sphincter cuff will be required. In boys the decision must be made whether or not to perform an external sphincterotomy so that the bladder can be emptied completely, following this with insertion of the artificial sphincter. An alternative approach is insertion of an artificial sphincter accepting that continued intermittent self-catheterization will be necessary. In girls, if the insertion of the artificial cuff alone does not make the child adequately continent then the pump and balloon will also need to be implanted.

Bowel function can be equally problematic in these patients. Assessment of anal tone is the key to management. If anal tone is weak, the child can only be continent of faeces if he or she is constipated. The problem then becomes one of emptying the bowel at regular intervals. This can be achieved by one of four main ways: straining, manual evacuation, suppositories or enemas. The frequency of emptying varies from child to child: between twice a day and once every two days. It is extremely unusual to have to resort to any radical means to treat faecal incontinence. If there is good anal tone, bowel emptying can usually be achieved by regular enemas and stress faecal leakage will not normally be a problem.

The management of bladder and bowel function does depend, to a large degree, on the cooperation and motivation of the patient. This is achieved with variable speed in spina bifida children.

Case 2

This 14-year-old boy has been referred from a 'distant place'. The boy has been wearing a suprapubic pressure device; an externally worn urine collection device which fits over the penis. He had to wear this because of continuous incontinence and enuresis. The boy walks satisfactorily although he has had to have several orthopaedic procedures on his feet and has some muscle wasting below the knees. His bowels are currently managed by straining after breakfast but he has some incontinence when he plays games at school.

On examination of the perineal area he has patchy loss of perineal sensation and some reduction of anal tone, although his anal reflex is present.

Questions

1 What is the likely diagnosis and cause of his incontinence?
2 How would you investigate him and what would you be likely to find?
3 How would you treat him?
4 What long-term problems may be experienced following definitive treatment?

Answers

1 In view of the findings of intact sacral arc fibres the micturition sacral reflex arc is likely to be, at least in part, preserved. This means that detrusor overactivity in the form of detrusor hyperreflexia will probably be present; however, as a reduction in anal tone was found urethral sphincter weakness is likely.
2 As this young man has had no supervised follow up, complete evaluation is necessary and this involves assessment of both upper and lower urinary tract. If the boy has had no recent contrast studies of the upper tract an intravenous pyelogram (IVP) would be sensible.

   Video urodynamics are used to assess lower urinary tract function but also give some other useful information, such as the presence or absence of vesico-ureteric reflux. However, the main information required from video urodynamics is an assessment of detrusor function both during filling and voiding and a similar assessment of the urethra.

   The results of the investigations in this young man showed normal upper tracts with prompt excretion of contrast medium on IVP into a bladder which showed the neuropathic picture of gross sacculation with a 'fir tree' outline. The urodynamics showed, on filling, some reduction of underlying bladder compliance with a gradual increase in detrusor pressure from 0 to 20 cm water. Superimposed on this reduced compliance were some phasic waves of detrusor contraction – detrusor hyperreflexia.

   The bladder was filled at 10 ml per minute without removing the residual urine at the start of filling. These points are important, as to empty the bladder or fill too fast, will produce quite marked alterations in the bladder and urethral activity that is normal for that patient. During bladder filling, genuine stress incontinence could be demonstrated when the patient was asked to cough or strain. The bladder neck and approximate urethra were open throughout filling with a prostatic urethral diameter increasing as the bladder filled. Contrast could be seen entering the prostate via the prostatic ducts – a common finding in patients shown to have static distal sphincter obstruction or detrusor–sphincter–dyssynergia.

Attempted voiding was by straining without any evidence of significant detrusor contraction. Although the bladder was filled to a reasonable volume of 350 ml the young man only managed to void 200 ml giving a residue of 150 ml. Throughout voiding the urethra could be seen to be narrow at external sphincter level, characteristic of static distal sphincter obstruction. The urodynamic studies showed that the young man had two causes for incontinence, i.e. detrusor overactivity and urethral sphincter weakness.

3   It is generally accepted that detrusor activity in a boy of this age, who will require sphincter surgery to achieve continence, cannot be controlled by drug therapy. This means that bladder augmentation or substitution will be necessary to produce an adequate volume bladder of good compliance.

The decision had to be made as to whether this boy should be treated by external sphincterotomy followed 6 weeks later by implantation of an artificial sphincter, accepting that he would have to self-catheterize to ensure bladder emptying after surgery. However, in this case, it was decided to do a 12 o'clock full length sphincterotomy from bladder neck to the most proximal part of the bulbous urethra. A 7 o'clock bladder neck incision from the right ureteric orifice to the verumontanum was also carried out. If this is not done then full bladder emptying may not be possible due to bladder neck closure towards the end of micturition. Six weeks after external sphincterotomy, end-oscopy showed the urethra to be healed and open, with full bladder emptying being achieved by straining. At this time through a midline incision an artificial sphincter cuff was implanted around the membranous urethra, i.e. below the prostate and above the pelvic diaphragm. At the same procedure the bladder was split in the coronal plane with the incision passing immediately anterior to the ureteric orifices. On incision of the bladder, the bladder muscle appeared healthy and not overly thick. A 20 cm segment of ileum was isolated, with its own blood supply, split along on its antemesenteric border, and inserted into the defect that resulted from bivalving the bladder. Continuity of the ileum was restored with a two layer catgut anastomosis and

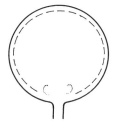
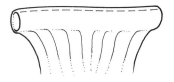

(a)

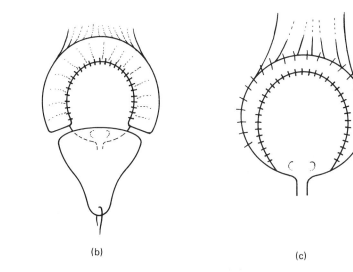

(b)

(c)

Figure 23 (a) The bladder is opened in the coronal plane and a 20 cm piece of ileum along its antemesenteric border. (b) One edge of the ileal segment has been sewn to the edge of the posterior part of the bladder. (c) The completed cystoplasty showing the ileum and its mesentery incorporated into the bladder

the mesenteric defect closed.

Implantation of the artificial sphincter cuff required division of the pubourethral and puboprostatic ligaments together with incision of the endopelvic fascia over obturator internus. This allows the surgeon to develop a plane between the rectum and the urethra using the urethrally placed catheter, and a finger in the rectum if necessary, to ensure neither the urethra nor rectum is transgressed. The tubing from the cuff was brought through the right rectus muscle into a pouch lying close to the mid-inguinal point deep to fat but superficial to rectus sheath. The patient was kept on 7 days of parenteral antibiotics (cefuroxime and metronidazole) and most importantly the bladder was flushed through the two catheters (urethral and supra-pubic) every 2 hours to ensure proper bladder drainage. This point is particularly important as the long suture line means that the new bladder cannot be watertight until healing has occurred. After one week the urethral catheter was removed and following a cystogram 2 weeks later which showed no leaks the supra-pubic one was removed, the patient going home with a condom external appliance for urine collection.

Six weeks later the patient was readmitted, when he was still incontinent, and had a minor operation through a transverse right inguinal incision when the artificial sphincter control pump was implanted into the right scrotum and a pressure regulating balloon, designed to give a sphincter cuff pressure of between 71 and 80 cm water was implanted via the inguinal canal and into the extraperitoneal tissues. Two days postoperatively the patient found the scrotum comfortable and it was therefore possible to activate the sphincter. The AMS800 artificial sphincter has an activation/deactivation button and when the sphincter was implanted it was implanted deactivated with the cuff empty and the fluid (dilute contrast medium) held in the balloon. When the sphincter is activated then, under pressure the cuff is filled from the balloon and urethra consequently compressed.

Over the next 24 hours the patient was taught to use the sphincter, initially every 2 hours. It required six pumps of the sphincter control device in the scrotum to empty the cuff and to transfer the fluid (0.5 ml per pump) to the balloon. Ultrasound examinations of the bladder showed that he was fully emptying the bladder. He was allowed home and followed in the outpatient department.

4   There is some controversy as to whether a sphincter should be implanted at the same time as a cystoplasty is performed. However, there is little evidence that there is any accompanying increased risk of infection of the sphincter. Infection of the sphincter is a significant problem in meningomyelocele and sacral agenesis patients, but this seems more related to whether they are patients who have previously suffered multiple urinary infections.

The later problems between the patient's discharge and say 12 months following surgery include urinary infections, problems with excess mucus production and difficulties with the artificial sphincter. Urinary infections, if they produce systemic upset, are evidenced by cloudy foul smelling urine, and should be treated promptly and adequately. If the patient suffers persistent infections then long-term low dose antibiotics are necessary. If the patient still gets breakthrough infections on low dose trimethoprim then it is useful to rotate monthly through four antibiotics such as nitrofurantoin, a cephalosporin, ampicillin, and trimethoprim. If infections are recurring the patient's ability to empty the bladder should be checked.

Excess mucus production can be a problem but the patients generally adapt to this. However, if there is blockage or difficulty voiding due to mucus then regular consumption of cranberry or black grape juice may help. An alternative recently suggested medication that seems successful is the use of the H2 blocker, ranitidine. The artificial sphincter is generally very reliable but some patients may experience problems and it is certainly worth checking the patient's technique. Some patients inadvertently deactivate the sphincter so that the sphincter is in the 'cuff empty' position leading to recurrent incontinence.

Long-term complications of these procedures may again be related to either the sphincter or the cystoplasty. Mechanical problems do occur with the sphincter and on occasions a leak may develop in the system which shows itself as recurrent incontinence. X-raying the patient may show that the system is empty, and it is then advisable to replace the whole system. Occasionally the cuff erodes into the urethra and very occasionally into the vagina or rectum. It may be that erosion only ever follows a chronic infection of the sphincter, however, it is almost always essential to remove the whole device. Reimplantation of the sphincter can occur after a suitable interval of at least 3–6 months. The long-term side-effects of cystoplasty are mainly concerned with the uncertainty that exists concerning the incorporation of gut segments into the urinary tract. It is known that ureterosigmoidostomies, an early form of urinary diversion, are accompanied by a significant incidence of neoplasia developing at the junction of the urothelium and the gut mucosa. Initially these are adenomas but they develop into adenocarcinomas.

Tumours have been described in cystoplasties but, in most cases, these patients have not been followed adequately, nor had proper treatment of urinary infection or adequate management of chronic residual urine, hence it seems very sensible to maintain patients with cystoplasty under close follow up with proper treatment of urinary infection and regular checks on the adequacy of their voiding. It is presumed that it will be necessary to commence check cystoscopy once a year to look at and biopsy any suspicious areas developing in the neobladders.

Case 3

This patient is an 18-year-old woman who had been diverted at the age of two years because of development of upper tract dilatation noted while under urological follow up in the spina bifida clinic. At this time she had a right iliac fossa ileal conduit. She led a normal life and had attended normal school despite her conduit. However, she had recently become unhappy, in body image terms, with her ileal conduit and asked whether she had to stay the way she was. On examination of the perineum she had excellent anal tone and the anal reflex was present. She was slim and the ileal conduit looked healthy.

Questions

1 Does this woman have to continue with her ileal conduit?
2 How could she be investigated?

3 How could she be managed?
4 Are there any current indications for formation of an ileal conduit in neuropathic patients?

Answers

1 As discussed in Case 1 it is now most unusual to form an ileal conduit since most patients can be managed by a combination of intermittent self-catheterization, anticholinergics, augmentation cystoplasty and artificial urinary sphincter. Hence, theoretically, this woman should also be manageable by such techniques. This philosophy has led to the development of techniques of 'undiversion'. In this woman's case the indication for undiversion is mainly social. However, in other patients, recurrent urinary infections due to conduit stasis, and stoma problems are medical indications for undiversion.

2 As in all problems of vesico-urethral dysfunction the primary aims of investigation are to define the function of the detrusor and urethra during filling and emptying, as well as the need to reassess upper tract function.

The passage of contrast medium into the ileal conduit will show whether or not there is reflux from the conduit into one or both ureters. In this woman's case there was bilateral reflux with prompt drainage of the contrast medium back into the conduit and out through the stoma into the drainage bag. An intravenous pyelogram showed good cortical thickness with no scarring or dilatation.

We believe that if such patients were not diverted in this situation, urodynamics would have shown reduced bladder compliance and static distal sphincter obstruction with high resting urethral pressures. Therefore we believe that cystoplasty is almost always necessary and do not subscribe to the American proposal that bladder distension over a prolonged period should be done in an attempt to increase the patient's own bladder capacity to acceptable levels. Urodynamic investigations in those who have undergone diversion are confined to an assessment of the urethra and our most useful test is the static urethral profile. Experience has shown that if the maximum urethral closure pressure is equal to or greater than 50 cm water then the patient will be continent following a cystoplasty, and will be able to empty using intermittent self-catheteriz-ation. This young woman's maximum urethral closure pressure was 72 cm water; the normal range in young women would be 50–85 cm water.

After investigation the patient was advised that un-

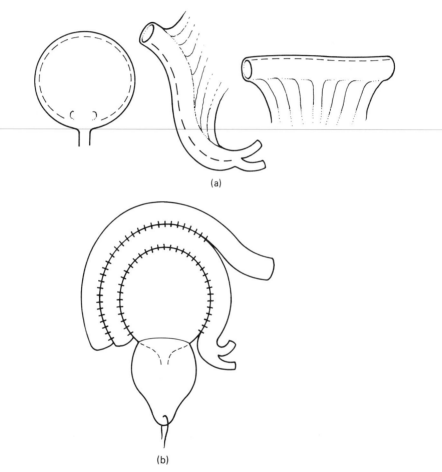

(a)

(b)

Figure 24 (a) The bladder is opened in its coronal plane and the ileal conduit and ileal segment along their antemesenteric borders. (b) The opened ileal conduit has been sewn onto the posterior bladder edge and the ileal segment is being sewn onto the other edge of the ileal conduit. The procedure will be completed by sewing the free edge of the ileal segment to the anterior wall of the bladder

diversion was possible with the use of a cystoplasty and intermittent self-catheterization.

3   In our experience undiversion should only be carried out after the most thorough counselling of the patient together with the teaching of intermittent self-catheterization *pre-operatively*. In this young woman's case undiversion is mainly for social reasons and clear consent must be obtained to perform such relatively major surgery for social reasons. Nevertheless we believe that these social reasons are extremely powerful and have been very gratified to witness the marked alteration in the psyche of patients who have undergone undiversion. The restoration of body image, in terms of ridding the patient of an external appliance, often produces very marked improvement in the patient's ability to deal with the world. Relative shyness and introversion are often replaced by a more smiling and open personality.

As intermittent self-catheterization is frequently needed it is essential that it is explained, taught and then performed by the patient prior to surgery. Once the patient is happy and skilled at the technique then surgery can go ahead.

This woman was well motivated to surgery and performed intermittent self-catheterization most efficiently. Through a mid-line incision, the ileal conduit was dissected, then detached from the skin and underlying tissue and pulled through into the peritoneal cavity. The bladder was opened in its coronal plane, the ileal conduit was split along the distal 12 cm of its length after excision of the skin end. A further 20 cm segment of small bowel was isolated on its blood supply and similarly split along its antimesenteric border. The ileal continuity was restored with a two layer catgut anastomosis and the mesenteric defect repaired.

One side of the opened ileal conduit was sewn to the posterior edge of the open bladder. The other edge of the opened ileal conduit was sewn to one edge of the new segment of ileum and the second edge of that ileal segment to the anterior edge of the bladder. As the bladder wall appeared quite healthy none was excised. The patient was left with a urethral and a suprapubic catheter, these were both flushed 2 hourly with saline to prevent mucus blockage and after 7 days the urethral catheter was removed.

At 10 days the patient was sent home to be readmitted 4 weeks from the time of operation for a cystogram to make sure there was no urinary leakage. This cystogram was satisfactory and the suprapubic catheter was clamped. The patient then started intermittent self-catherization and after 24 hours was happy with the technique. The suprapubic catheter was removed and after a further 12 hours the patient was allowed home. The only antibiotics given were for 24 hours over the period of the operation.

Certain findings during investigation would have changed the way in which this young woman was managed. Had the upper tract studies shown dilatation and no reflux in the ileal conduit then the ureters would have been re-implanted into the cystoplasty using an anti-reflux technique such as the Le Duc method. Had urodynamics shown that the maximum urethral closure pressure was less than 50 cm H_2O then an artificial sphincter cuff would have been implanted. In the female the cuff is implanted at the junction between the bladder and the urethra and the plane between the vagina and the urethra is found by exposing the white vaginal tissue in a similar way to the technique used during colpo-suspension. The para-vaginal tissues are swept off the vaginal finger to reveal the white extra-vaginal fascia. It is then possible to pass an instrument beneath the urethra and create a tunnel wide enough to implant the sphincter cuff. In females the implantation of the cuff alone often results in adequate continence. In order to prevent erosion either into the vagina or into the urethra the omentum is mobilized from the transverse colon and, if necessary, either the left or right gastro-epiploic artery is divided to give extra length. The omentum is then split and a part is put between the cuff and the vagina and another part between the cuff and urethra – an 'omental sandwich'. Had the bladder been obviously thickened and diseased then the bladder would have been excised down to the bladder neck and a full bladder substitution performed, rather than a bladder augmentation.

4   An ileal conduit is still occasionally indicated. The chief indication is in patients who are quite markedly deformed by associated skeletal deformities such as those seen in spina bifida. These may result in the patient's chest and upper abdomen resting on their knees as they move around in a wheel chair. With such severe skeletal deformities

it may be relatively awkward for the patient to transfer from a wheelchair onto an ordinary toilet to perform self-catheterization or to void. Recurrent urinary infections and gross sphincter weakness necessitate major urethral surgery and in such patients may push the management towards an ileal conduit. In these circumstances an ileal conduit may come as a great relief to the patient and make their lives considerably easier.

It is particularly important to place the stoma carefully on a convex easily accessible part of the abdomen free of skin creases. This usually means in the upper part of the abdomen, not too close to the rib cage and well away from the umbilicus.

Case 4

This 25-year-old male patient has suffered from life-long nocturnal enuresis. He has never been free from this problem and complained that he wet the bed at least five nights each week. In the daytime he had urinary frequency voiding 10 times each day despite restricting daily fluid intake to approximately 1 litre. On the nights when he did not wet the bed he woke and passed his urine in the middle of the night. On occasions he also had daytime urge incontinence losing small amounts into his underwear but rarely did this come through onto his outer clothing. He complained of social restriction due to this problem and in particular found it very difficult to go to the pub in the evenings with his friends and consume any quantity of beer or lager. If he did then he would have marked frequency and urgency and would have to avoid going to bed until very late in order to void most of his alcohol intake and prevent wetting the bed at least twice during the night. As he was a long distance lorry driver his daytime frequency was also inconvenient.

On examination there were no physical abnormalities to find.

158

Questions

1 How do you imagine this patient has been treated in the past?
2 How would you investigate him now?
3 What are the causes of enuresis?
4 How would you manage his problem?

Answers

1 Formerly, enuresis was felt to be a largely psychological problem. In the 'bad old days' children with enuresis were certainly beaten repeatedly and faced social ostracism. In more recent times their therapy has been based on less judgemental attitudes. This young man had been treated by behavioural therapy in the form of star charts: a system of rewarding the child for dry nights. He had also tried a bell and buzzer on two occasions. The bell and buzzer is a device where the child sleeps on a pad containing wires connected to a battery. If the pad becomes wet the wires become shorted and a buzzer sounds. This is a form of behaviour therapy probably based on lightening the child's sleep and making him aware of the fullness of his bladder. Unfortunately in this man's case one month's period of treatment with a bell and buzzer was unsuccessful. He was also tried on imipramine at night and this too proved unsuccessful. Imipramine has local anaesthetic effects, anticholinergic effects and central depressant effects. Although it is successful in many patients with enuresis it was not successful in this patient.

2 In view of the fact that this man had had previous treatment he was investigated by urodynamic testing. His urine flow rate was excellent with a maximum flow rate of 42 ml per second for a voided volume of 250 ml and no residual urine. Urodynamics showed a markedly unstable bladder although he did not leak during the test. His sphincter function was normal and he had a high maximum urethral pressure of 100 cm water (normal range is 60–100 cm water). His plain abdominal X-ray was scrutinized but there were no skeletal defects such as spina bifida occulta and his sacrum was intact excluding sacral agenesis.

3 There is controversy regarding the aetiology of enuresis.

It is certain that the patients who have daytime urgency, urge incontinence and night-time enuresis have a very high incidence of detrusor instability which must be implicated in the production of these symptoms. However, approximately 50% of patients have no daytime problems and are merely enuretic. The relatives of such patients claim that they sleep very deeply and, particularly during trials of the bell and buzzer, everybody in the house wakes up except the patient. Hence there seems to be some association with deep sleep. Enuretic patients have been shown to have a reduced cystometric and cystoscopic capacity and therefore a small bladder also appears to contribute. The last mechanism recently discovered is that many enuretic children and young adults fail to concentrate their urine normally at night and will pass more than one-third of their 24-hour urine production during the sleeping hours.

4　An understanding of the pathogenesis of enuresis helps in its logical treatment. If detrusor instability is a factor, as in this patient, then treatment with anticholinergic drugs may help. The use of oxybutynin (5 ml three times a day) or probanthine (15–30 mg three or four times a day) by day, with or without imipramine 25 mg taken in the evening may be effective. As this man had not had an adequate trial of anticholinergic therapy a combination of oxybutynin and imipramine was tried. Despite pushing the dosage up until he developed a dry mouth (anticholinergic side-effect) his night-time symptoms in particular were not helped. A course of DDAVP (desmopressin, an ADH anologue) was taken intranasally and in this patient an initial dosage of 10 μg was tried. This was unsuccessful and was raised to 20 μg. This improved his enuresis considerably although he was still wet at least twice a week. Unfortunately there was little effect on his daytime symptoms as he had been unable to tolerate anticholinergics. A decision was made that conservative treatment of his daytime and night-time problems had failed.

In view of the limitation on his social and working life that his bladder problems caused, he wished to have further treatment.

Ileo-cystoplasty ('clam' cystoplasty) is currently viewed as the only successful means of treating such patients. In the last 20 years, various denervations have been attempted, including sacral neurectomy, cystolysis (where the bladder is separated from all extra-vesical tissue until the whole bladder has been skeletalized apart from the urethra and ureters), bladder transection (both endoscopic and open) and injection of Phenol or other injurious substances around the ureteric orifices. Despite promising early results from these denervation techniques, at 2 years most reports show a recurrence of the patients' original problem. Hence denervation procedures have been largely abandoned in favour of the 'clam' cystoplasty. After discussion with this patient an ileocystoplasty was performed. The technique was identical to that described in Case 1.

Postoperatively this patient did very well and was cured of his daytime and night-time problems. He is currently under surveillance to ensure that he empties his bladder properly and to monitor upper tract function and the presence or absence of urinary infection.

Case 5

This 30-year-old man while on holiday in the 'Costa Packet' had, after a long night's drinking, gone down to the seashore and dived off some rocks into the sea. Unfortunately the tide was out and he dived into only 2 feet (60 cm) of water. He sustained a fracture dislocation of the low cervical spine and became tetraplegic. After initial care he was transferred back by air ambulance to the UK.

He arrived with an indwelling catheter and in an obviously shocked and emotional state. On examination he was found to have a C7 sensory level. Hence he had good function of his shoulders but some reduction of function in his forearms and loss of fine movement in his fingers. He had no reflexes present below the level of his cord transection and hence was thought to be in the stage of spinal shock.

His immediate management consisted of providing psychological support, he required manual evacuation of his bowel and his urinary catheter was removed, his bladder being emptied regularly by sterile intermittent catheterization by the nursing staff.

Questions

1 What further investigations should be performed?
2 How will he be managed in the next 6 months from the urological point of view?
3 What options does he have for voiding?
4 What should be his long-term urological care?

Answers

1 Once there is some return of reflex activity for example, the anal reflex or leg spasms, then urodynamic tests should be done. After 8 weeks he had a slow fill cystometrogram which showed reflex bladder activity at a volume of 300 ml. The detrusor contractions were small and poorly sustained, resulting in some voiding and a residual urine of approximately 200 ml. An intravenous pyelogram (IVP) was also performed at this stage which was normal.
   At 12 weeks slow fill urodynamics were repeated and he was shown to have a good detrusor contraction at 350 ml that resulted in complete bladder emptying.

2 Once reflex bladder activity has returned then the patient can be rehabilitated from the urological point of view. In this man's case, reflex bladder activity could be triggered by suprapubic tapping. The patient was taught to tap firmly in the suprapubic area a dozen times at intervals of 2 seconds. This successfully stimulated a detrusor contraction and the patient was able to void into a bottle which he held himself. He could achieve this sitting in the wheelchair that he had been taught to use. By watching his fluid intake and tapping his bladder every 2 hours he was able to be dry only 6 months after his accident. He had also been taught to regulate his diet and to do manual evacuation to empty the bowel.

3 In this man suprapubic tapping, stimulating reflex bladder contraction was initially successful. However, at follow up 9 months after injury, the patient reported that the volumes voided were diminishing and, he had had several incontinent episodes. In view of this the urodynamics were repeated which showed the onset of classical detrusor–sphincter–dyssynergia (Figure 25). Sphincter dyssynergia is common in patients with high spinal cord injuries. It

is characterized by phasic contractions of the urethral sphincter during reflex detrusor contractions. This results in an interrupted urine flow, eventual fatigue of the detrusor and significant residual urine. This man's residual urine had increased from 0 to 150 ml. In this case an alternative option had to be sought. The choice was between teaching the patient intermittent self-catheterization together with the use of anticholinergic drugs to increase his functional bladder capacity, or the performance of an external sphincterotomy to render him completely incontinent which would necessitate urine collection by an external applicance. The patient opted to be taught intermittent self-catheterization and successfully learnt this

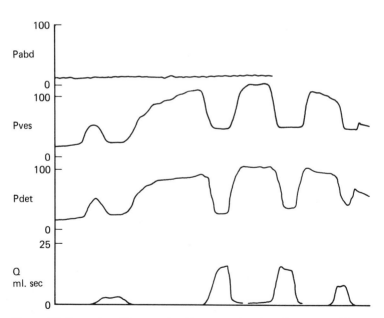

Figure 25 Expand voiding cystometrogram showing detrusor–sphincter–dyssynergia. The reciprocal rise in flow rate (Q) with a fall in pressure (P_{det}) is due to the sphincter being open during the periods of flow but closed in between. Pressure rises in the absence of flow because the detrusor is contracting against a closed sphincter. Intra-abdominal pressure (P_{abd}); Intravesical pressure (P_{ves})

technique despite the fact that his hand movements were limited. As he was not completely dry on intermittent self-catheterization, oxybutynin 5 mg three times a day was added and he regained full continence.

Many patients opt for an external sphincterotomy as they find it easier, being wheelchair bound, to have a condom catheter appliance draining into a leg bag worn under their trousers. This frees them from the need to go to a toilet at regular intervals and certainly allows them to go out drinking with the 'lads'. The external sphincterotomy ensures full bladder emptying at the price of complete incontinence.

Other options for bladder drainage include the use of an indwelling catheter. While this is generally discouraged, it is not thought to be as harmful in the long term as previously believed. However, close supervision of the patient would be necessary if this option was chosen. A construction of an ileal conduit is rarely indicated in the paraplegic patient as most are males and can be managed by one of the means already discussed.

The sacral anterior route stimulator (SARS) is a recent innovation which is highly promising. The use of the stimulator demands the existence of an intact sacral micturition reflex. In these circumstances, via a lumbar approach, the sacral nerve routes can be dissected out and their dorsal components cut. Stimulating electrodes are put onto those anterior root nerves which are shown to be motor to the bladder. Connecting wires from the electrodes run up onto the anterior chest wall to the receiver. By using a transcutaneous stimulator the sacral nerves can be stimulated and micturition produced. This technique can also be used to achieve penile erection and sometimes defaecation.

If a patient has previously had a sphincterotomy and wishes to be dry then this can only be achieved by insertion of an artificial sphincter, and voiding by regular tapping or by intermittent self-catheterization.

4   The long-term follow up of paraplegic patients is extremely important. Urinary infection and renal stone formation were the cause of the deaths of most paraplegic patients up to the end of the Second World War. This situation was revolutionized by the introduction of sterile catheterization at Stoke Mandeville Spinal Injury Unit. Despite this innovation, it is still essential to follow patients carefully and regu-

lar assessment of the upper and lower urinary tract is needed. Detrusor–sphincter–dyssynergia can develop at any stage following injury, as can upper tract dilatation. Hence 6–12 monthly ultrasound tests of the upper tract and the bladder for residual urine are mandatory. In patients with long-term catheters there is an increased risk of stone formation and stones must be dealt with promptly and efficiently.

Case 6

A female patient aged 45 with a 10-year history of multiple sclerosis was referred because of urological problems. The patient had complained of incontinence and had been treated for recurrent urinary infections with courses of antibiotics. On interrogation the patient was voiding urine every 1–1.5 hours during the day and was having to get up twice at night. Her urinary frequency was due to urgency and on occasions she failed to get to the toilet and leaked. This necessitated the use of three medium-sized incontinence pads per day. On occasions, despite an urgent desire to void, when she arrived and sat on the toilet she was unable to pass urine. Her referral had been precipitated by the recent onset of 12 episodes of enuresis. The urinary infections she suffered were often slow to clear and required more than one course of antibiotics; she had had four attacks of infection in the preceding 6 months.

On examination she walked reasonably well with the aid of a stick. She had suffered some loss of manual dexterity. Examination of the lower limbs revealed brisk reflexes. There were no abnormalities on examination of the perineum and no demonstrable incontinence on coughing.

Questions

1 What is the likely cause of this woman's problems?
2 What investigations should be performed?
3 What treatment could be instituted immediately?
4 What are the long-term urological problems of multiple sclerosis?

Answers

1   The symptoms of urgency and urge incontinence are very strongly suggestive of detrusor overactivity; in this case detrusor hyperreflexia. Failing to void despite an urgent desire suggests failure of urethral relaxation and in multiple sclerosis this is due to detrusor–sphincter–dyssynergia (see Case 5). The history that urinary infections proved hard to treat suggests the possibility of residual urine, stone or resistant organisms.

2   Urinary tract ultrasound would reveal upper tract dilatation and any urololithiasis in either the upper or lower urinary tract. Upper tract dilatation is unusual in multiple sclerosis despite being common in other forms of neuropathic vesico-urethral dysfunction. In this patient no abnormality was found. A mid-stream urine (MSU) showed significant pyuria with 60 white cells per high power field and a pure growth of *Escherichia coli*. She was treated immediately with a full course of antibiotics, her urine checked and, when found to be clear, video-urodynamics were performed.

The urodynamics showed an unstable bladder on filling, with urge incontinence. The lower urinary tract appeared normal in outline on the video film. At capacity of 280 ml she developed extreme urgency and the filling catheter was removed to allow her to void. The video showed that the bladder neck was open but the urethra closed at sphincter level.

After a period of 40 seconds the sphincter relaxed to allow the passage of some urine but the detrusor contraction was poorly sustained. The urethra closed and, after a further period, a second wave of detrusor contraction produced another minor void. She had a residual urine of 220 ml. Her initial residual urine had been measured by ultrasound at 150 ml. (Note: as with other patients with neurological disease, her bladder was not emptied at the beginning of urodynamic testing and was filled at 10 ml per minute.)

3   As suspected from her history this woman's problems were of detrusor overactivity during filling, together with a functional outflow obstruction due to urethral overactivity during voiding. This problem was approached initially by teaching the patient intermittent self-catheterization.

Despite some limitations of hand movement she achieved this quite rapidly and was able to catheterize herself 2-hourly. However despite this, at her next review in the clinic after 6 weeks she still reported annoying episodes of urinary incontinence. In view of the finding of detrusor hyperreflexia she was then treated with oxybutynin 5 mg three times a day. This produced a very satisfactory response. She became dry and reduced her frequency of catheterizations to 2.5–3-hourly depending on the volume of fluid she drank. In future her dose of anticholinergic will be varied according to her need and if possible she will try to manage without drug medication. However, it seems unlikely she will be able to manage without performing intermittent self-catheterization.

In this case, because of the history of recurrent infections the patient was treated with low dose trimethoprim for the first month of self-catheterization. However, once the antibiotics were stopped she had remained free of infection when last seen in the outpatient clinic.

4 The problems of detrusor overactivity and urethral overactivity illustrated by this woman's findings are typical of MS patients. Not all patients can be managed in this relatively conservative way and at present there is a developing discussion about early aggressive management for this condition. This discussion has been hampered in the past by the fluctuating nature of the disease with its remissions and relapses. However, it seems certain that the bladder does not improve sufficiently to free the patient totally from treatment once the symptoms have developed.

If anticholinergic therapy is insufficient to control the detrusor overactivity then 'clam' cystoplasty may need to be considered. Intermittent *self*-catheterization is a slightly misleading term in that with small children and the elderly or handicapped, the catheterization can be done by the carer and this is certainly true for patients with multiple sclerosis. It is arguably easier for a carer to catheterize an MS patient than to have to help that patient change their wet clothes and bed linen with the attendant waste of time and expense on laundry.

The other option that could be considered is that of diverting the urine to an ileal conduit. Once again it may be easier for the carer to manage an ileal conduit with its external appliance than to manage repeated episodes of incontinence.

If the patient becomes markedly disabled and eventually suffers a loss of muscle power necessitating the permanent use of a wheelchair or even becomes bed bound, then the urological problems can become compounded. We have many patients in our clinics who have been managed for many years with indwelling catheters and they tend to develop a patulous urethra which cannot exert an adequate closure pressure and hence the patient not only has incontinence secondary to detrusor overactivity but also to urethral sphincter weakness. These two conditions often cause leakage around the catheter and while this has been improved by using catheters of small calibre with balloons of only 5 ml, significant incontinence may persist. This problem can be approached in a number of ways. First by the use of a suprapubic rather than a urethral catheter hence moving the catheter balloon away from the trigone the bladder may be stimulated to contract less frequently. However this does not answer the problems in every patient and the operation of urethral closure has been devised in conjunction with suprapubic catheterization as the next step in management. This operation is technically quite difficult and best done by a combined perineal and supraubic approach; it is best done by specialist hands.

Case 7

This man of 55 years of age was referred to the clinic because of a 5-year history of urinary difficulty. He complained of a slow stream and hesitancy. In addition to these symptoms he was voiding 2-hourly by day and rising once from his bed to pass urine at night. He had noticed no incontinence and no other worrying symptoms such as haematuria. He was otherwise fit and on examination his prostate felt smooth with moderate enlargement. The central and lateral sulci being felt easily.

On closer interrogation he also complained of difficulty of voiding in the presence of others and of leaking at the end of micturition.

Questions

1 What is the differential diagnosis in this man's case?
2 What investigations would you organize?
3 What treatment would you consider in this man's case?
4 What alternative treatments exist for the treatment of bladder outflow obstructions in male patients?

Answers

1 Working from basic principles, urine flow must be related to other expulsive forces of micturition which consist of detrusor contraction and abdominal straining, and the retentive forces which include the mechanical and functional aspects of urethral activity. Mechanical aspects would include prostatic obstruction or urethral stricture and functional aspects would include the smooth muscle activity of the urethra and the striated muscle activity of the external sphincter and pelvic floor. Hence it can be seen that low flow may be due to an obstruction, either mechanical or functional, or to poor expulsive forces such as seen in a detrusor underactivity, or indeed to a combination of obstruction and detrusor underactivity. This man finds himself at the beginning of the prostatic age group when some 20–30% of the male population have a prostate ultrasound volume of greater than 20 ml.

The other symptom which bothered him was hesitancy and this symptom may again represent either outlet obstruction or detrusor underactivity. In outlet obstruction, because a higher pressure is required to open the urethra, micturition onset is delayed for several seconds for the same detrusor contraction. Similarly if the detrusor is relatively underactive then the patient will have to wait to start voiding.

For the sake of argument, if you assumed that this man's problem is due to outlet obstruction then the obstruction may be anywhere from the bladder neck to the tip of the penis. Bladder neck obstruction is relatively unusual and may represent either a functional abnormality, that is the bladder fails to relax or a mechanical obstruction where there has been contraction of the bladder neck elements. Numerically prostatic obstruction is the commonest cause of blockage, although urethral strictures at any level are frequently seen. It should not be forgotten that a meatal stricture can also give a reduction in urine flow and can be easily diagnosed on physical examination.

2   This man should have basic urological tests which include either a plain abdominal X-ray of the abdomen or an ultrasound of the abdomen and this is designed to look for bladder or kidney stones and may well pick up a significant residual urine assuming the patient has been asked to void immediately prior to the investigation. Similarly a midstream urine specimen should be sent to the laboratory for examination of cells and for urine culture. Some patients with bladder cancer can mimic outflow obstruction although this man's symptoms would not suggest this. If in any doubt a urine cytology should also be performed to exclude carcinoma in situ of the bladder as a cause of the patient's symptoms.

Intravenous pyelography (IVP) was thought to be mandatory but a recent metanalysis has shown that the IVP is not a useful investigation in outlet obstruction. Similarly, while endoscopy of the lower urinary tract is valuable in excluding other pathologies such as stone or tumour it is not useful in determining whether the patient has an outlet obstruction with the sole exception of the diagnosis of the urethral strictures. Urethrography would be an alternative acceptable means of looking for a urethral stricture.

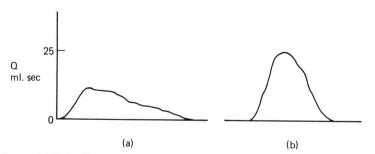

Figure 26 Urine flow readings preoperatively (a) showing a maximum flow rate (Q_{max}) of 11 ml/s compared to a Q_{max} of 25 ml/s postoperatively (b)

The definitive test for bladder outlet obstruction is the pressure flow study of micturition. During these urodynamic tests the pressure within the bladder and rectum are measured throughout filling and emptying. During emptying the urine flow rate is also measured. In classical outlet obstruction high pressure is accompanied by low flow: there may not be a residual urine. A man of 55 should void with a flow rate of greater than 15 ml per second for voided volumes in excess of 150 ml. The maximum detrusor voiding pressure should be less than 50 cm water. In this man's case his maximum flow rate was 11 ml per second and his detrusor pressure maximum flow was 90 cm water. He had a small residual of 100 ml having had his bladder filled to 400 ml. Incidentally urethral pressure profilometry, which is the measurement of the pressure within the prostatic urethra has certain features which correlate well with the presence of obstruction as judged by high pressure flow studies. The length of the prostate and the height of the prostatic plateau, that is the pressure exerted by the lateral lobes of the prostate on the measuring catheter also correlate significantly (Figure 27).

3   This man, after full discussion elected to have a transurethral resection of his prostate (TURP). At endoscopy no other cause for obstruction such as a urethral stricture was found and a 25 g transurethral resection of prostate was carried out uneventfully. Postoperatively he was delighted

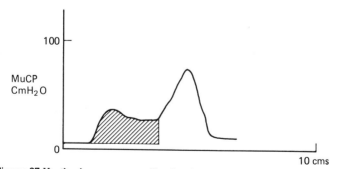

Figure 27 Urethral pressure profile showing the area (hatched) which represents the prostate and disappears after a full resection of the adenomatous tissue

by the results of surgery and a follow up mid-stream urine (MSU) demonstrated that there was no infection. His urine flow rate postoperatively had increased from 11 ml per second to 25 ml per second.

4 TURP remains the gold standard in the treatment of prostatic obstruction. It is an excellent procedure with good relief of symptoms, at least in patients without extensive coexisting disease such as chronic respiratory or cardiac vascular problems. Nevertheless, a number of alternative techniques have emerged in the last 10 years. First drug treatment. Drug treatment of outlet flow obstruction is proceeding along three lines. In the prostatic capsule and bladder neck and prostatic tissue itself there are large numbers of alpha-adrenergic receptors and hence alpha-adrenergic blocking drugs have been developed to relax the bladder outlet. Indoramine and Prazocin are marketed in the UK for this purpose. They have a moderate action improving flow rates and symptoms by some 30%. However this margin can be sufficient to make some patients happy to carry on without surgical intervention. More recently there has been an effort to find drugs that actually shrink the prostate and these drugs consist of five alpha-reductase inhibitors and aromatase inhibitors. These drugs are responsible for blocking the conversion of testosterone into dihydrotestosterone (DHT) and androstenedione to oestrogen respectively. DHT is largely responsible for prostatic growth and oestrogens have a significant trophic effect on stromal tissue. As yet it is too early to say whether these new modes of treatment will be as successful as alpha-adrenergic blockade.

Balloon dilatation of the prostate has been developed over the last 5 years and this has a similar effect to alpha-adrenergic blockade in improving symptoms and flow rates in about 30% of patients. This can be used in the younger male patient who wishes to avoid prostatectomy because of its attendant problem of retrograde ejaculation.

Cryosurgery to the prostate has been used in the past for treating elderly patients and has been moderately successful in the treatment of retention of urine. More recently there has been extensive interest in hyperthermia to the prostate. This technique involves a passage by either rectal or urethral probe into the area of the prostate and then heating the prostate area using microwaves. As yet we have no objective evidence to show relief of outflow obstruction by prostatic hyperthermia, however, there seems to be an appreciable improvement in the patient's symptoms. The last novel treatment for a prostatic obstruction is the use of internal prostatic stents. Stents are available made of gold, stainless steel and titanium (Figure 28). These can be placed either under radiological or endoscopic control into the prostatic urethra so that they extend from the bladder neck to the prostatic apex. These are intended for use in elderly patients who have significant coexisting disease making them a higher risk for prostatic surgery. The early results of prostatic stenting are favourable with the majority of patients being freed from indwelling catheters. It is likely that prostatic stenting will have a permanent place within the urological armamentarium.

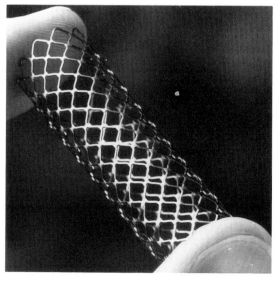

Figure 28 The ASI titanium prostatic stent

Case 8

A 59-year-old woman has been referred to the clinic with a 10-year history of increasing urinary incontinence. The patient complains that she leaks on a daily basis requiring the use of four incontinence pads during the day but none at night. She reports that her leakage occurs if she coughs or sneezes but also that leakage occurs if she fails to get to the toilet in time. She was voiding every 1.5 hours during the day and getting up once at night. She is a married woman and has had three normal deliveries.

On examination she is a moderately obese woman weighing 70 kg and her height was 163 cm (5′ 4″). There are no abnormalities on examination of the abdomen but on examination of the perineum, after asking the patient to cough repeatedly, urine leakage occurred. There is also some descent of the anterior vaginal wall on coughing and straining.

Questions

1 How should this patient be managed initially?
2 If initial management fails to cure the problem how should she be investigated?
3 What are the pathophysiological processes that might cause incontinence in a woman of this age?
4 What surgical procedures are available to treat this type of patient?
5 How do you choose which procedure to perform?

Answers

1 From this woman's history the presumptive diagnosis of stress incontinence can be made. However, a detailed history should be taken and by the end of a symptom analysis it should be clear to the clinician whether or not the patient is suffering from symptoms that could be mainly explained by stress incontinence or by urge incontinence. In this woman's case, although she has got some urgency it is quite clear, from her history, that most of her leakage is due to stress events such as her coughing, stumbling,

lifting heavy objects etc.

A variety of conservative measures can be used in the treatment of presumed stress incontinence.

First from examining the woman any evidence of oestrogen deficiency should be sought. If atrophic changes are seen then an oral or vaginal course of oestrogens for 2 months should be prescribed.

The other measures that can be adopted to treat the patient conservatively in the initial phase are aimed at reducing the general factors which worsen stress incontinence. Continence in general and stress incontinence in particular depends on maintaining the differential between urethral pressure and bladder pressure – the urethral closure pressure. Obesity and other factors that raise the intravesical pressure reduce the urethra closure pressure and exacerbate incontinence. This woman was moderately obese and was therefore asked to lose 10 kg in weight. She was given dietary advice and an explanation that a combination of reduced food intake and increased exercise would be the quickest way in which to achieve weight loss was happily accepted by her. She was not a smoker but had she been she would have been asked to give up smoking prior to her operation. There is little scientific evidence that losing weight or stopping smoking reduces stress incontinence. However, it is certainly commonly accepted by many clinicians specializing in the treatment of incontinence.

Pelvic floor exercises represent the other significant area of conservative management. If the patient can contract her pelvic floor at times of 'stress' then incontinence may be prevented. Unfortunately many women, like our patient, have lost the ability to contract the pelvic floor at will. The strength and efficiency of the pelvic floor should be assessed during the vaginal examination, asking the patient to tighten her pelvic muscles as if she was drawing up her pelvic floor or trying to interrupt her urine stream while voiding. When asked to do this many women will contract their buttocks and abdominal muscles. It needs to be carefully explained that contraction of these muscles and in particular of the abdominal wall muscles will tend to raise the bladder pressure and make incontinence worse rather than help prevent leakage. If the patient is able to contract her pelvic floor then a scheme of pelvic floor exercises is given to that patient. These consist of asking the woman to perform a series of contractions. It is our practice to ask the woman to initially contract her pelvic floor for 5 seconds relaxing it for 5 seconds and repeating that contraction 10 times. The patient is asked to do 10 sets of 10 contractions each day. When she is able to contract her pelvic floor for 5 seconds then she extends that to 10 seconds and she is thereafter doing 100 contractions for 10 seconds each day. She should be encouraged to maintain this level of pelvic floor exercise for at least 2 months.

If the woman is unable to contract her pelvic floor then a number of 'tricks' are available to teach her to do so. Perineometry is a method of measuring vaginal pressure. A tube-like device connected to a pressure gauge is passed into the vagina and lies across the pelvic floor. The patient is asked to try various manoeuvres until she finds the one which increases the pressure registered by the perineometer while not involving abdominal muscle contraction. Pelvic floor faradism is an electrical technique whereby a stimulating electrode is put into the vagina and the ampage and voltage increased until the patient's pelvic floor is made to contract by the electrical stimulation. By this means it is hoped that the patient learns to contract her pelvic floor and goes on to do pelvic floor exercises.

Intravaginal cones are a relatively new method of exercising the pelvic floor (Figure 29). They are supplied in a

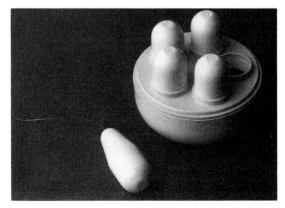

Figure 29 Plevnik weighted vaginal cones for pelvic floor exercises

series of five cones, of identical size, but of differing weights. The cone has a tail of nylon from its pointed end and it is inserted blunt end first into the vagina. In order to prevent the cones slipping out, onto the floor, the patient has to use her pelvic floor muscles. As in ordinary pelvic floor exercises the patient is encouraged to hold the cone for a longer period, and when she can successfully do this, the next cone, i.e. the next heaviest, is used for the same set of exercises.

Whichever methods are used to treat the patient conservatively it is wise to wait at least 2 months prior to further investigation and management.

2 In view of the patient's persistent leakage urodynamic studies were carried out. These consisted of uroflowmetry, pressure flow measurements during voiding and both static and dynamic urethral pressure profilometry. These investigations showed her to have a stable bladder with demonstrable stress incontinence at volumes greater than 150 ml. She was able to hold 380 ml and voided to completion after removal of the filling catheter. She demonstrated a rise in detrusor pressure of 15 cm water during voiding and had maximum flow rate of 28 ml/s. Her static urethral pressure showed a maximum urethral closure pressure of 36 cm water and a functional urethral pressure of 2.5 cm.

Hence urodynamics had shown this woman to have genuine stress incontinence secondary to a reduction in pressure transmission to the urethra.

3 Unfortunately after 3 months, despite having lost more than 10 kg weight, this woman was still significantly incontinent requiring, on average, three pads per day. She expressed a desire to have definitive treatment as her incontinence caused her quite significant social limitations. As she had had no previous surgery, she was treated by an endoscopic bladder neck suspension (Stamey procedure). She was admitted on the day of operation and under general anaesthesia the Stamey procedure was performed. This involved two small vaginal incisions in the anterior vaginal wall either side of the bladder neck, and two small suprapubic incisions 2 cm lateral to the mid-line and two fingers' breadth above the upper edge of the pubic symphysis. Using long Stamey needles no. 2 nylon sutures were passed on either side of the bladder neck to form two

loops. The loops were prevented from cutting through either at the vaginal end or the rectus sheath by 1 cm long silastic tube buttresses. By endoscopy, the correct positioning of the needle at the junction between the bladder neck and urethra was ensured. Similarly endoscopy checked that the needle had not transgressed the bladder. Should the needle enter the bladder at any stage, the needle is withdrawn and passed again. When the nylon loops were in place, the vaginal incisions were closed with chromic catgut. The loops were then tightened in order to elevate the vagina behind the pubic symphysis on either side of the bladder neck. The suprapubic incisions were closed and the suprapubic catheter inserted. The patient spent the next day resting and on the second postoperative day was sufficiently mobile for the suprapubic tube to be clamped. She quickly established normal voiding with no residual urines and at the end of the second postoperative day the catheter was removed and she went home. She was advised not to do any heavy lifting or severe exertion for 3 months.

4   You may not have chosen to do a Stamey procedure on this patient and it must be immediately accepted that other procedures are widely performed. Other procedures can be divided into three groups.

Firstly, vaginal procedures have been the traditional gynaecological operation for genuine stress incontinence (GSI), the best known being the anterior repair (Kelly operation). In this operation excess anterior vaginal tissue is removed and the remaining anterior vaginal wall brought across to the mid-line thereby providing better support for the urethra. In this procedure, efforts are made to approximate the cardinal ligaments at bladder neck level in order to support the bladder neck further.

Secondly, combined suprapubic and vaginal approaches. These operations have become the standard in treating GSI. The Stamey procedure represents a simple form of combined operation as do the Raz procedure and the Gittes procedure. Each of these procedures depends on the passage of a long needle through the rectropubic space to secure a suture from the vagina to the anterior rectus sheath, either side of the bladder neck. The Burch culposuspension procedure is perhaps the gold standard of procedures for GSI. The principle of this operation is to suture the anterior vaginal wall to the back of the pubis on either side of the bladder neck. Hence the vaginal wall, between these two points of attachment, provides a hammock supporting the proximal urethra and bladder neck region. The anterolateral vaginal wall is elevated and sutured to the back of the pubis. As a long suprapubic incision is required for this procedure the patient's recovery tends to be slower and the patient needs to stay in hospital for up to 7 days.

Thirdly, sling procedures have been tried for many years but have a bad reputation partly due to their propensity for producing voiding dysfunction and their tendency to erode through the urethra. In these procedures a sling of either natural or artificial material is passed around the bladder neck and suspended on either side from the anterior rectus sheath. The chief reason for their bad reputation is because they are used in circumstances where the patient has very poor urethral function and following one or more previously failed procedures. The sling is used to compress the urethra and is normally put in under some tension. It is this tension which probably results in the erosions and voiding problems. It is likely that sling procedures can be used effectively using less tension and hence preventing erosion. Although sling procedures have been done in a few male patients the artificial urinary sphincter represents the best chance of continence for male patients with sphincter weakness leakage (see Case 5).

5 Genuine stress incontinence is due, in part at least, to two main factors. First, malpositioning of the bladder neck/ urethral junction and secondly intrinsic urethral sphincter weakness. These two main factors govern the choice of procedure.

In women who have had no previous surgery the anterior vaginal wall and bladder are usually fairly mobile. Hence one's surgical endeavours are usually directed towards repositioning of the bladder neck. In patients who are neurologically intact this procedure is usually sufficient to ensure cure. However, if there is an element of denervation, such as in women or girls with myelomeningocele, then repositioning of the bladder neck may not be sufficient and it may be necessary to perform either a sling procedure or to implant an artificial sphincter.

In women who have had previous bladder neck surgery then there may be fixation of the bladder neck to the anterior vagina and it will be necessary, prior to any reposition technique, to mobilize the bladder base and proximal urethra from the underlying scar tissue in the anterior vaginal wall. This can be done by an inverted 'U' incision in the anterior wall and the interposition of a labial fat pad (Martius technique) between the bladder neck/ proximal urethra and the anterior vagina. If there is poor urethral function as evidenced by a low urethral closure pressure (less than 20 cm water) then it may be wise to perform either a sling procedure, a Stamey-Martius procedure or the insertion of an artificial sphincter. However, the position has been somewhat complicated by the advent of intramural urethral collagen injections. This technique seems to have an excellent short-term cure rate in patients who have rather fixed bladder necks and low urethral closure pressures.

Case 9

This 78-year-old man was referred from a distant place having undergone a transurethral resection of the prostate (TURP) for benign prostatic hypertrophy 2 years previously. Prior to that operation he had gone into acute retention and had reported slow stream and hesitancy together with some urgency prior to the retention episode. The operation had been difficult and complicated by heavy blood loss. Following removal of his catheter 5 days after surgery he was incontinent. Despite teaching of pelvic floor exercises his incontinence persisted and he had to wear incontinence pads. These pads proved unsuccessful and he developed excoriation of the external genital and groin regions. He was then converted to wearing a condom type urinary incontinence device. He was reasonably satisfied with this device for some period although it would fall off at inopportune moments creating considerable inconvenience and social embarrassment if he happened to be out of his home. On examination, this man was very fit for his age and in the habit of walking 3 km (2 miles) twice a day. There were no neurological features.

Questions

1 What are the possible causes of incontinence in this man's case and which of these is the most likely?
2 How should he be investigated?
3 How should he be treated?
4 What other conditions may cause incontinence in elderly male patients?

Answers

1 This man's incontinence dates from the time of his prostatic surgery. His original prostatectomy had been for a urinary retention and hence the presence of postoperative retention and associated overflow incontinence had to be, and was, excluded by the clinicians looking after him.

Prior to operation he had had some urgency at micturition and indeed had had occasional urge incontinence. Hence detrusor instability would have been a possible cause of his leakage. However, his leakage was often not related to any feeling of urgency.

The most likely cause of incontinence with this symptom history, would be peroperative sphincter damage during TURP. This was particularly likely in this case as the man's prostatectomy was complicated by heavy bleeding. On close questioning he said that his leakage was worsened by walking and by being generally physically active. It was this factor that led him to seek further treatment, in view of his liking for long walks.

2 The investigation of choice following simple investigations such as plain abdominal X-ray, and urine to exclude infection, would be video urodynamics. As well as inflow and voiding cystometry urethral pressure profilometry was carried out. During filling cystometry he did show some unstable detrusor activity which on one occasion produced a small leak. The video showed that his bladder neck was widely open and a sizeable prostatic fossa was visualized. He was asked to 'heel bounce' that is, to lift himself up and down on the soles of his feet. During this movement he could be seen to leak in the absence of any detrusor contraction. Hence genuine stress incontinence (GSI) was confirmed. The appearance of the urethra was

smooth. The urethral closure pressure was 15 cm water. However this is much less than the normal values of 50–100 cm water. Urodynamics had confirmed GSI secondary to sphincter weakness incontinence due to sphincter damage during TURP.

3   After discussion this man elected to have a perineal artificial sphincter implanted. After ensuring his urine was sterile this sphincter was implanted via a mid-line perineal incision. He was readmitted for 24 hours 3 weeks later for sphincter activation, managed the sphincter easily and was discharged home to be followed up in outpatients.

4   The commonest cause for urinary incontinence in elderly men is bladder overactivity (detrusor instability). Detrusor instability is found, during bladder filling, in 50% of men over the age of 70 and becomes even more common in the very elderly infirm. It is likely that the increasing incidence of detrusor instability is secondary to subtle brain changes and research has shown that there are sub-clinical brain changes on MRI and dynamic brain scanning. While many patients with detrusor instability have no apparent cause, with increasing age, the incidence of conditions such as stroke, senile dementia and Parkinson's disease becomes

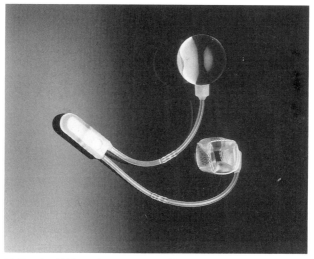

Figure 30 The AMS800 artificial urinary sphincter

higher. All these conditions lead to a high incidence of bladder overactivity and consequent incontinence.

So called 'overflow incontinence' usually accompanies a high pressure chronic retention. Characteristically, an elderly man will report that he has begun to wet the bed during his sleep. Examination of the abdomen usually reveals an enlarged tense bladder and if ultrasound is carried out, his upper tracts will usually be dilated because of a back pressure effect on the kidneys. Such patients do well from outflow tract surgery (TURP).

Stress incontinence in the elderly man is extremely unusual and usually only follows, and is due to, surgery such as TURP.

Case 10

This 83-year-old woman was referred from a nursing home where she was presenting considerable problems in view of her incontinence. She had been admitted to the home following a cerebrovascular accident from which she had made a good recovery but, insufficient to allow her to continue living alone in her home. Her admission to the nursing home had been 2 years previously and in those 2 years she had suffered some deterioration of cerebral function becoming somewhat forgetful and occasionally confused.

She came to the clinic accompanied by a care assistant and it was difficult to establish a pattern of her leakage from the history given. The patient did not realize she was incontinent and the incontinence did not seem to trouble her.

On examination she was slightly confused and disorientated in time and place. She was moderately obese and on examination of the abdomen the colon was readily palpable. Inspection of the introitus revealed atrophic changes to the vulva and perineum. On rectal examination she was found to be faecally impacted.

Questions

1 What are the likely causes of this woman's incontinence?
2 What investigations should be performed?
3 How can she be treated?

Answers

1 The three most likely causes of incontinence are first detrusor hyperreflexia secondary to her cerebrovascular accident and dementia, secondly, stress incontinence secondary to urethral sphincter weakness, and thirdly overflow incontinence secondary to her faecal impaction. In the elderly, urinary infection can cause symptoms identical to those of detrusor instability.

2 In the elderly institutionalized patient urodynamic investigations are now rarely carried out. The main reason for this is that findings tend to be predictable, with detrusor instability as the prime cause of incontinence. As in any other branch of medicine, no investigation should be done if the results are easily predicted.

Hence investigations should be pragmatic and in this woman a catheter was passed to obtain a clean specimen of urine. This failed to show any urinary infection but did show a residual urine of 100 ml. A plain abdominal X-ray was done to exclude conditions such as a bladder stone which might be producing her symptoms.

3 In this woman, treatment of her faecal impaction had a high priority; the lower bowel was cleared with enemas and she was put onto a higher roughage diet.

At the same time, she was given topical oestrogen cream which was applied by the nursing staff in the home. Similarly barrier creams were used to try to reverse the skin changes found in the perineum. The nursing and care staff were asked to take her to the toilet on a 2-hourly basis.

She was fitted with proper pads and pants and while in bed a rewashable incontinence sheet was used to protect the bed clothes.

Her progress was slow and because her incontinence was not fully controlled she was tried on a course of anticholinergic treatment: oxybutynin 2.5 mg three times per day.

Her progress continued and the skin condition stabilized. She remains somewhat incontinent but is more adequately managed by the techniques now employed. Several random post void catheterizations have shown that she no longer has a residual urine. The problem of detrusor hyperactivity in the elderly with chronic retention has recently been highlighted and is well treated by intermittent catheterization by the family or carers if patients are not capable of this themselves.

Index